Nursing Stories

New Directions in Anthropology

General Editor: **Jacqueline Waldren**, *Institute of Social Anthropology, University of Oxford*

NURSING STORIES

Life and Death in a German Hospice

Nicholas Eschenbruch

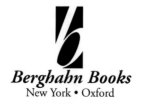

Berghahn Books
New York • Oxford

First published in 2007 by

Berghahn Books

www.berghahnbooks.com

© 2007 Nicholas Eschenbruch

Library of Congress Cataloguing-in-Publication Data

Eschenbruch, Nicholas, 1972-
    Nursing stories : life and death in a German hospice / Nicholas Eschenbruch.
      p. cm. -- (New directions in anthropology ; v. 27)
    Includes bibliographical references and index.
    ISBN 1-84545-151-1 (hardback : alk. paper)
      1. Hospice care—Germany. 2. Hospices (Terminal care)—Germany.
    3. Death—Social aspects—Germany. I. Title. II. Series.

RT87.T45E83 2006
362.17'560943—dc22   2006017173

British Library Cataloguing in Publication Data

A catalogue record for this book is available from the British Library.

Printed in the United States on acid-free paper.

ISBN 1-84545-151-1 hardback

CONTENTS

PREFACE

Death, which concerns all people, is a classical topic of anthropology. Individuals and social groups in all cultures and societies develop strategies to integrate death in their way of seeing the world, and of living in the world as they interpret it. Not surprisingly, however, there is great historical and cultural diversity in the explanations provided for death, in the social arrangement of its exact circumstances, in the ways of dealing with the changes it causes and in the literature which various academic disciplines have contributed to the study of death and dying.[1]

This study is about illness, dying and death in a German hospice, about lives lived, things done and stories told there. Against the backdrop of a large German city, it shows how a number of people – patients, nurses, relatives, an ethnographer and others – deal with dying and death in a model institution specifically created for that purpose. Of central concern is the question as to how meaningful experience is constructed for terminally ill patients, based on distinct notions of the person a patient is, by encouraging specific ways of approaching social interaction and living daily life. Based on fieldwork in nursing care, primarily as a participant observer, the analysis focuses on the interaction of patients and nurses in routine, everyday situations and looks at the underlying values, attitudes and assumptions within such interaction.

Concerning its genre, the present text is an ethnography. Ethnography, through participation and observation, generates specific knowledge from within the social practices it describes, linking personal experience of the minute details of everyday life with analytical tools and theoretical concepts from the academic domain, and reflexively monitoring this process. Ethnography uses the analysis of the particular to elucidate the very general aspects of the human condition, as temporary and precarious as the results must always remain. Much of its value lies in the creative tension resulting from the inherent contradiction.[2]

In this sense, the present study will not only describe hospice life in detail from an ethnographic perspective, but also combine such description with a discussion of some very general anthropological questions. Resulting from the hospice nursing experience and woven into the account of it are several perspectives of methodological and theoretical relevance for anthropology, culminating in a specific view of ethnography as a participatory method for interpretative social research in one's own society, and in a corresponding perspective on conceptualisations of death.

During the course of the study, I will take up some of Michael Carrithers' ideas (1991, 1992, 1995, in press) and take a close ethnographic look at stories, especially 'minimal narratives' (Carrithers 1995: 268). Furthermore, I shall argue that narrative patterns of interaction and communication, called 'therapeutic emplotment' by Cheryl Mattingly (1994, 1998), are an essential means in nurses' attempts to construct meaningful experience for patients in their last weeks. I will then draw this together to suggest the self-reflexive use of narrative as a coherent method for participant observation in highly involving fields, especially for anthropology 'at home'.

Also, based on arguments about personhood originally laid out by Anthony Giddens (1991), extended to the study of death and dying by Tony Walter (1993, 1994) and taken into the British hospice context by Julia Lawton (2000), I shall comment throughout on the relations between narrative, death and contemporary ideas of the person. Finally, drawing all these strands together, I will use the idea of 'absolute metaphor', as introduced by German philosopher Hans Blumenberg (1998[1960], 1971), contextualise it for anthropology with James Fernandez' (1986) work on metaphoric predication, and thus arrive at a unified theoretical view of the ethnography of death in contemporary Western societies.

Ethnographic scholarship about medicine, nursing, death and dying in these societies is not a uniform venture. While this study does not identify with one specific trend or current of anthropological thought, but rather attempts its own approach, I am of course indebted to a number of fields of research on which such an approach necessarily needs to be built. British Sociology, first of all, has set the methodological and especially theoretical standards for all later hospice research. This is especially true for the work of Tony Walter (1991, 1993, 1994) and the fine, more recent study by Julia Lawton (2000). Also Clive Seale (esp. 1998) and various collaborators have set standards.

However, all their research took place in Britain and is set in the context of the NHS, an encompassing institutional structure indeed. I needed to bear in mind the specific German cultural and institutional framework of my own research, a context in which, for one thing, there seems to be more flexibility regarding institutional culture in hospices than in Britain. The only ethnographic study of a German hospice that I could consult throughout the time of my research was Christine Pfeffer's book (1998), which focuses on interviews, mainly with hospice nurses.[3]

My writing is also informed by approaches associated with, mainly North American, medical anthropology. However, I am not so certain that such a general label for an already heterogeneous field really fits my own work, and some such influences, while definitely present, are quite indirect.[4] Finally, as only became fully apparent to me after the first typescript was finished, I have also been influenced by a not so likely ally, Donna Haraway (1988, 1997). Her understanding of metaphor, narrative and reflexivity, and more so her own use of these devices and perspectives, has been important for my thinking and writing.

In spite of this variety of influences, and while sociological theory and statistical surveys on death, dying and the hospice movement now abound, there are still quite few detailed ethnographic studies of death and dying in contemporary Europe. Mulkay and Ernst have pointed out that 'We can encompass the full historical and cultural variability of people's conduct in relation to death only if we consistently supplement the conventional, medically defined concept of "biological death" with a sociological concept of "social death"' (1991: 195). In addition, I argue, we will also have to get a close ethnographic picture of the social realities in which both concepts of death are played out and from which they have both emerged. To provide one such picture is the aim of the present study.

The first chapter will introduce key concepts for the anthropological analysis of death and dying and will provide background information for the hospice movement. The second chapter is devoted to developing the methodological framework for the following ethnography. Chapter three provides a detailed ethnographic documentation and discussion of daily nursing practice in the hospice context and looks at its values and assumptions. Chapter four shows how narrative structures are important in the negotiation of meaning, hope and social interaction in the hospice. Chapter five is concerned with actual deaths and the practices and stories surrounding them. Chapter six provides a summary and conclusion of the whole study and presents further theoretical results for the discipline of anthropology.

Notes

1.   Generally speaking, there is now more literature in this field than one person can work through. To make matters more complicated, some of this literature, both in German and English, is situated in a grey zone somewhere between the social sciences, advice books for the terminally ill and their relatives, esoteric thought, and nursing textbooks, with an often curious mixture of all of these elements. Many such books, while they are without doubt very valuable for some audiences, add little theoretical and methodological insight from an academic point of view. I have thus been quite selective in my references and do not attempt to give a complete list of the literature pertaining to my topic. I apologise if I should have overlooked relevant publications. The two classical theoretical essays relevant for the study of death in anthropology are still van Gennep (1986[1909]) and Hertz (1928a). The standard introductory works providing a theoretical overview of the anthropology of death and presenting several detailed case studies are Huntington and Metcalf (1991[1979]), and Bloch and Parry (1982). The standard historical synthesis is Ariès (1997[1978]) who is, however, at times exceedingly romantic about death in the past, as criticised e.g. by Elias (1985: 23–29) and Armstrong (1987). Two relatively recent,

book-length sociological introductions are Seale (1998) and, in German, Feldmann (1997). For overviews of the older literature, see Simpson (1987[1979]), Southard (1991), Kan (1992), Wiedenmann (1992) and Walter (1993).

2. I shall come back to this at greater length in chapter 2. Some of the authors who have been influential for my understanding of ethnography are Geertz (1995[1973]), Flick (1998[1995]), Spradley (1980), Lindner (1981, 1988, 1995), Turner (2000) and Hirschauer (2001).

3. More recently, the German Federal Hospice Working Party (Bundesarbeitsgemeinschaft Hospiz, BAG) has become active in publishing and, due to their efforts, the ethnographic position of my own study can now be supplemented by a survey of hospice care in Europe (Gronemeyer et al. 2004), a brief quantitative overview of nurses' work situation in German hospices (Schröder et al. 2003) and three collections of short articles sponsored by the BAG (Bundesarbeitsgemeinschaft Hospiz 2004a, 2004b, 2004c). A more recent monograph-type study on hospice care in Germany is Gerstenkorn (2004), a theological dissertation analysing twenty interviews with nurses from three hospices, mainly in a framework of professionalisation theory. Christine Pfeffer's second sociological study of hospice care in Germany (Pfeffer 2005), based on several years nursing experience in hospices, and Stefan Dreßke's monograph (Dreßke 2005) came out after this manuscript was finished. Julia von Hayek is presently completing a study on non-residential hospice care. All three are recommended, but could not be considered anymore for my own argument in this book. Kirschner's (1996) first-ever study of a German hospice is still empirically valuable.

4. Byron Good (1994) and Deborah Lupton (2003[1994]) provide informative overview accounts of social studies of biomedicine. See also Kleinman (1988), Berg and Mol (1998a, 1998b) and the contributions to Albrecht et al. (2000).

ACKNOWLEDGEMENTS

Like any such project, this study came into being in a web of social relations, and I would like to acknowledge those who contributed to it in many significant ways: First of all, I thank everybody at Stadtwald Hospice for bearing with me and teaching me a lot about life and death. I am still very grateful. I also thank Harald Haury, who followed the project from day one and provided essential encouragement and constructive criticism throughout. At Humboldt University's Institute for European Ethnology in Berlin, feedback and support were given on many occasions by Alexa Färber, Corinna Henning, Christine Holmberg, Bettina Sebek, Franka Schneider, Anja Schwanhäußer and Victoria Schwenzer. Peter Niedermüller supported my research from the start and very reliably provided precise analyses, important institutional backup and subtle criticism. Stefan Beck was quick and encouraging when an additional evaluation of my work was needed in its final phase. Michael Carrithers at Durham University gave decisive theoretical input and pulled out the right book from the shelf at the right time more than once. Working with him was a great and lasting inspiration. Ulrich Tröhler and my colleagues in Freiburg provided a congenial working atmosphere in which to prepare the first draft for publication. When it came to preparation of the final typescript, the help of Nadine Metzger was invaluable. Most important, however, was the support of my family in all those times when future developments were yet uncertain. The Studienstiftung des deutschen Volkes made the whole project possible with a research grant for which I am very grateful, and it is through the efforts of everybody at Berghahn Books that the result of that project is now in front of you. All mistakes remain my own.

This book is dedicated to the memory of Wolfgang von Buch, who encouraged me.

1
APPROACHES TO
HOSPICE DEATH

Perspectives on 'Dying'

Anthropology, according to James Fernandez (1986: xi),[1] begins with 'revelatory incidents' and ethnography proceeds through personal encounters. One such encounter, revealing in a brief incident a lot of hospice life, was part of my longer nursing relationship with Hans Dornschuh. When I met Hans, I was working as an assistant nurse in a hospice institution for the terminally ill in a large German city – I shall refer to it as Stadtwald Hospice. I was working there for the purpose of doing ethnographic fieldwork and, since that is probably not a fully sufficient explanation for me being there, I was also working there for the personal purpose of finding out something about death.

Hans was in his early sixties when he became a hospice patient because of his lung cancer. He had spent a good deal of his life in a closed psychiatric ward because of a psychosis somehow related to the untimely death of his daughter. A somewhat rough-looking, extremely charming man, Hans flirted with any nurse who would come and talk to him, called male nurses his smurfs or his little mice and wanted and gave a lot of physical contact and affection. Everybody called him by his first name. In spite of his cancer, which by then had become very severe, tied him to his bed and forced him to inhale oxygen at regular intervals, Hans continued his heavy smoking habit. This is one of my diary entries about him:

Tonight, Hans gets oxygen most of the time, in between he rings regularly. Then, the same scene happens every time: I enter his room, say hello Hans, Nicholas my little one he says, then takes my hand or my arm and strokes it a little, how are you, Hans, I ask,

1

then one of us makes some joke, Hans has a good sense of humour considering his situation, and then he says, somewhat shy, mate, will you switch off the oxygen and open the window, I laugh and say Hans, you don't want to smoke again, do you? He smiles and protests, it's been only one pack today, I used to smoke two and a half. I open the window widely, switch the oxygen off and light him a cigarette. Hans sometimes smokes when he is on his own, which worries the nurses because of the fire hazard. I sit with him, we chat a little, Hans smokes cigarette-sized cigarillos, which he inhales. He already breathes heavily and smoking is very tiring for him. Most of the time he cannot finish the cigarillo, then he needs oxygen again and starts breathing in gasps and with a rattling sound. So I switch the oxygen on again. An hour or so later, he will call me again, and the scene will be repeated.

My story about Hans is a good starting point for all that follows because it very well illustrates hospice life as I experienced it: devastating illness coexisted with a great determination to make life worth living, in an atmosphere of care and accompanied by a hearty disregard for many rules normally characterising biomedical institutions. Quite significantly, also, death can only be found in the story by extrapolation and by a speculative extension of the story line into the future. There is a characteristic paradox here, which will run through the whole study: while any hospice situation is, ultimately, about death, hospice practice turns out to be mainly about life.

The notion of dying is the mediating category between the two. In the German hospice context, where the central concern of hospices and hospice work is seen to be '*Sterbebegleitung*' ('death accompaniment'), the term 'dying' is almost ubiquitous.[2] The whole hospice idea rests to no small extent on this notion, which by itself, as Julia Lawton points out, is rather unsatisfactory to explain the existence and function of hospices anywhere (2000: 145). I take 'dying' as the analytical point of departure for drawing up a conceptual framework, because my ethnographic work with people like Hans Dornschuh was placed in a temporal space delineated by it and in a semantic space implied by it.[3]

The term 'dying', as Sudnow (1967: 64) has already noted in his classic study of death in two American hospitals, is essentially a predictive term. It postulates an outcome, death, and thereby asks for a positioning towards that outcome by patients, other people concerned and larger social groups. It also postulates a trajectory in time, waiting to be filled with a plot. In many ways, 'dying' is a call to action for parties thus far uninvolved in a patient's life: once death and the time that precedes it are drawn together into the temporal and normative unit of 'dying', delineated by biomedical definitions and based on biomedical authority, they can be made the subject of intervention by hospices, palliative care units, therapists and, ultimately, social scientists.

Such a dying phase of life now exists independently of awareness by any individual patient. On the contrary, it is assumed to exist prior to patients' awareness. This is, for example, shown by the fact that there is a widely discussed research issue of patients being 'informed', 'unaware' or 'in denial' of their dying situation

(Armstrong 1987, Seale 1991, Seale et al. 1997). In a similar vein, those who direct their efforts toward living the rest of their lives as normally as possible have been labelled 'heroic' (Seale 1995) – the ascriptions seem inescapable. All this confirms that there are specific activities and attitudes expected of the dying person, activities and attitudes which differ from the regular social repertoire and owe their existence to the notion of dying: 'when subjects are seen to be dying those with whom they come into contact respond by seeking to impose a special frame of reference in terms of which further interaction is to be organized' (Mulkay and Ernst 1991: 174).

If we are all mortal, however, why are some people labelled as 'dying' and others not? Due to the development of modern biomedicine and its increasingly accurate diagnostic methods, it is possible today to refer to people as 'dying' as soon as a physician states that there is no possibility for further curative biomedical treatment of a severe illness.[4] A starting point of a dying phase, and of the social role of the dying person that comes with it, is thus primarily defined by biomedical authorities. It is based on their specific biomedical knowledge which in turn rests, at least to a large extent, on epistemological categories and methods of verification deemed valid in the natural sciences. Such a point of view is not necessarily universal or undisputed – my emphasis on the biomedical view here is owed to the hospice nursing perspective. From that perspective, a patient entering a hospice is known to be dying and has been biomedically labelled as such, regardless of whether she herself or her relatives think the same way.[5]

Just as the entry into a dying phase is marked by biomedical authorities, so is the exit, namely death. Again, closer inspection reveals that death is far from being an obvious biological occurrence, and the question as to what death actually is merits closer attention. Intuitively, death may seem something blatantly clear, a fact of nature, the only future event in our lives of which we can be absolutely sure. However, while this may be so, recent empirical studies in the history, sociology and anthropology of medicine all suggest that there is no one point at the end of life that can be defined as death by reference to some unchanging fact of nature.[6]

Whatever criterion is chosen to mark the onset of death – cessation of the pulse or respiration, lack of neuronal activity, or the like – it is always subject to negotiation concerning both its initial formulation and its diagnostic implementation. In fact, the more sophisticated the chosen criterion becomes in biomedical terms, the more it will depend on the interpretation of images, measurements and data. In the case of brain death, such interpretation is sometimes strikingly at odds with the perceived evidence of direct sense impression: a beating heart and a breathing person. While death has undeniable power over all that lives, as an ascription of a status on a body it still remains a social matter. An objective determination of the moment of death is impossible, even for the most objective science. From this point of view, there is no biological death outside the social.

How can such an insistence on the primacy of the social in defining death be reconciled with the indisputable fact that we all die and cannot deconstruct our end away? Philosopher Thomas Macho (1987) argues that it is in principle wrong to confuse any category of clinical death, based on biomedical diagnosis, with death itself, which can only ever be ascertained retrospectively. Macho, in a wide-ranging study of philosophical, anthropological, biomedical and literary contributions to the topic, convincingly shows that the term 'death', understood not as a designation for some negotiated point in time but as the very antithesis to life, cannot have a concrete reference.

Macho goes on to suggest that death can, however, be understood as a metaphor, an empty metaphor of which it cannot be said precisely what it is it substitutes for (Macho 1987: 181–83). He bases this argument on philosopher Hans Blumenberg's work on the role of metaphor in language, and especially in the history of philosophy and science. Blumenberg suggests that we use irreducible metaphors, which he calls 'absolute' metaphors, in order to capture aspects of thought which are beyond strictly logical reasoning, or, often in a vaguely prescient way, at the pre-rational base of such reasoning (Macho 1987: 188, Blumenberg 1998[1960]: esp. 8–13, Blumenberg 1971). He argues that such metaphors cannot be replaced by more direct or less equivocal terminology and ultimately concludes that language will forever escape attempts to structure the meaning of its terms in a strictly logical fashion.

In this sense, Thomas Macho suggests that we use images from other domains of thought and experience to fill out the experiential and cognitive void designated by 'death', which can never be filled philosophically, or by the natural sciences, but still persists as a deeply relevant and real element of our lives. There can be no strict rationality in any discussion of death: 'Our discourse about death cannot be demythologised. The mythical, metaphorical character of the term death in its daily usage is its *only meaning*' (Macho 1987: 183).[7] Any discussion of death is an interpretative discussion.

It is worth linking the philosophical inroad made by Blumenberg and Macho to the more ethnographically applicable thought of anthropologist James Fernandez (1986), because such linkage promises new perspectives not only on theory, but also on method. In a move similar to that of Blumenberg, Fernandez argues that metaphor is at the base of human thinking, but illustrates his argument with examples from social life rather than philosophy.

Especially, Fernandez proposes that anthropologists consider the notion of 'the inchoate', which he variously defines as 'a gnawing sense of uncertainty [...] which lies at the heart of the human condition and which energises the search for identity through predications' (1986: ix–x) or, more formally, 'the underlying (psychophysiological) and overlying (sociocultural) sense of entity (entirely of being or wholeness) which we reach for to express (by predication) and act out (by performance) but can never grasp' (1986: 235). Human beings, according to Fernandez, can ultimately never be sure who they are and what the world is. They resort to metaphorical designations to understand the central, but ultimately inchoate aspects of existence.

It is not so important for our present purposes to engage in a critical analysis of these definitions of the inchoate, which the author himself characterises as necessarily preliminary. What is more important is that Fernandez suggests a method as to how human beings deal with the inchoate and aptly illustrates it in a range of ethnographic contexts. This method is metaphoric predication, the designation of some aspect of experience by reference to another domain of our lives. Fernandez argues for his ethnographic material what Blumenberg states for the history of Western thought: at essential points, thinking resorts to metaphor.

Thus, we come to a point where a synthesis of Fernandez, Macho and Blumenberg can be attempted with reference to death: there are central, inchoate aspects of human life which are existentially highly relevant, continue to fascinate us deeply but forever escape rational inquiry. We can make them available in thought, communication and social life only by metaphoric predication, that is, by figuratively identifying them with elements from other domains of our experience with which we are more familiar. Death is one such central but inchoate aspect of our existence; we keep trying to define it and to pin it down through metaphorical operations which ultimately always refer us back to other aspects of our lives.

The referral to other aspects of life, however, also offers a way out of the dilemma: to pay attention to it is the only way to go on exploring the meaning of death – not by asking for a precise reference, which will forever elude us, but by enquiring how the term is employed, which images are used to cloak it with and how it relates to other metaphors and concepts which are used in its vicinity. This was already observed by Thomas Macho: why do we assume, for example, that metaphors of journeys and departure are meaningful in relation to death; why 'has he left us?'. Or, for the purposes of this study, what does death have to do with hospices beyond the potentially superficial observation that people die there?

In the course of this book, I shall expand on this question, illustrate it ethnographically and argue that metaphoric predication easily extends into narrative projection when a metaphor becomes a story. In order to do so, however, I will first take a closer look at the general ways death is dealt with in contemporary Western societies.

Social Death in Contemporary Life

Whatever the theoretical or philosophical perspective on death may be, in contemporary Western societies, as has been pointed out above, it can only be ascertained legitimately by a doctor. Biomedicine constitutes the most powerful discourse which makes it possible to attribute the status of 'dying' to some patients. Under different criteria, any or no human being could be called dying

5

and, in fact, some patients at the hospice in which I did my fieldwork lived longer than some of the staff. Especially in the case of cancer, patients often still have many months, sometimes years, to live when they are diagnosed as 'dying', and the time span between the abandonment of curative treatment and death is increasing due to further developments in non-curative medicine, such as palliative chemotherapy. 'Dying' has thus been a phenomenon of increasing occurrence and, as will be shown, has triggered an enormous amount of concern.

One reason for this is that biomedicine, in sharp contrast to its decisive role in the demarcation of dying, had less and less of a role to play within the dying trajectory. With growing diagnostic precision, it outlined an area of its own lack of power. The resulting emergence of a protracted last phase of life outside the reaches of curative medicine is an important precondition for the rise of the hospice movement. It is, however, not in itself sufficient to explain hospice values and motivations. An additional factor to be considered is that death poses a particular kind of challenge to the ideology of individualist, self-reflexive and self-responsible actualisation of biographies prevalent in the educated classes of Western Europe today.[8]

Contemporary life has been portrayed as a continuous process of designing, adapting and discarding individual drafts of biography and self-narrative. The self is seen as the responsible author of its own biography, past and future, the ideological assumption being that internal and external factors allow (or should allow) the person to be such an author, at least in principle. The present as the decisive moment of biography creation and redirection becomes the most important reference point of such projects. As Bauman (1992: 51–87) discusses in detail, such lifestyle ideology undermines all traditional possibilities to entertain ideas of continuity after death, be it through one's professional achievements, one's family or one's religious beliefs. In fact, putting such emphasis on the present, on change and choice, questions all possibilities for continuity as such. Mellor and Shilling (1993: 413) also point out that a great contemporary emphasis on the idealised youthful body makes it particularly difficult to integrate old age and death in conceptualisations of person and biography.

How does a lifestyle ideology of youthfulness, continuous self-actualisation and biographical redirection influence approaches to death and dying, and how does it deal with the appearance of a clear limiting horizon for any further projects? The most obvious seeming reaction is to maintain the dominant cultural practices of self-reflexivity, choice and individualism as long as possible. Modern individualism leads to the question as to how one can, as an individual, die one's 'own' way, in the same way one has – supposedly – lived one's 'own' life. This is where I see the most important ideological root consideration of the hospice movement.[9]

The circumstances of severe illness and the adversities of deteriorating health do, however, pose severe restrictions for dying one's own way. I shall come back in greater ethnographic detail to the physical limitation cancer imposes on the terminally ill. From a very practical point of view, self-actualisation and biography design are taxing, if not impossible, tasks for anybody suffering from progressing cancer, for whom the routines of everyday life present themselves as insurmountable obstacles. Personal independence usually comes to an end, and the ill person has to rely on others. Walter (1994: 189) has perceptively pointed out that one's own death, as advocated by the hospice movement, may be possible, but only in the company of others. This is the crucial practical starting point of the hospice movement.

In addition, the pursuit of self projects or the summarising of one's biography often become impossible through the loss of meaningful social contacts, or the inability to maintain them, long before biological death occurs. Sociology has introduced the term 'social death' for this phenomenon. Mulkay and Ernst, in a critical appraisal of earlier ethnographic work, suggest defining social death as 'the cessation of the individual person as an active agent in others' lives' (1991: 178). The notion can be illustrated most convincingly with reference to nursing homes for the elderly, where many live for years without any meaningful social contact at all, being totally limited to eating and excreting, not living their 'own' life, not dying their 'own' death, irrelevant for others. Social death, it has to be noted, by no means excludes dependency on others and contact with them, but these others are just not socially significant.[10]

The notion of social death is useful for this study because it helps to outline what I consider, drawing on Seale (1998: 7–8), to be the central aim of the hospice movement: social death must not occur before biological death, because it ends people's ability to continue an autonomous, self-reflexive and aware lifestyle. In the hospice view, patients must be given the opportunity to continue such a lifestyle against the adversities of deteriorating health, if necessary with the help of specifically designed hospice institutions. These are meant to support patients in dying their own way, in the company of others who help, maintaining as many social relationships as possible.[11]

A Brief Outline of the Hospice Movement

The hospice movement originated in the late 1960s in the United Kingdom and in the U.S. in close connection with a number of the discursive conditions and social developments outlined above. Taking a strong stance against a supposed 'denial of death' by society as a whole, and sometimes accusing the biomedical establishment of being inhumane and overly technical in orientation, the hospice movement made it its aim to enable terminally ill patients to live a self-determined, dignified last phase of life. For such patients, the hierarchical organisation and technical outlook of curative biomedicine were to be replaced by a patient-centred, self-determined and team-oriented approach, leaving a lot of space for patients' personal preferences in care and for the continuation and development of social relationships. Since hospice patients had no hope for cure anyway, curative medicine was to be replaced by palliative medicine, which focuses on the alleviation and control of unpleasant symptoms of disease, such as pain, vomiting or itching.[12]

Hospice institutions came to play a very prominent part in the early development of such palliative treatment. Hospices, by including other professional groups apart from medical doctors, were also designed to be more favourably disposed to physiotherapy, logotherapy, different forms of psychotherapy and alternative medicine than classical hospitals. From the beginning, the hospice movement placed considerable emphasis on 'meaning making'; the Christian religion, psychology and, later, esoteric New Age influences were a strong undercurrent amongst its proponents, and there is a vociferous Tibetan Buddhist minority in the hospice movement as well. All this certainly has to do with the fact that the central purpose-giving hope of biomedicine, the healthy body, is a powerless category in terminal care. Corina Salis Gross (2001: 29) points out that there is a close connection between the denial-of-death thesis, discussed below, and meaning-making, since death denial is usually described as resulting from a lack of meaning in death, which in turn is seen as a consequence of medicalisation and of the loss of importance of religious models of life and death.

The term 'hospice' was borrowed from medieval European institutions, to which writers from within the hospice movement like to trace back its roots. Today, the term is used to refer both to groups of volunteers visiting patients at home and to full-time nursing institutions, looking after patients twenty-four hours a day, seven days a week, with full-time staff, on their own premises. In both English and German, proponents of the idea will also sometimes use 'hospice' without an article or other qualifier, as a sort of abstract noun referring to an attitude or set of practices and ideas, as in a sentence such as, 'generally speaking, hospice aims at empowering patients'.

Two women are widely considered the founding figures of the hospice movement and the most prominent reference points in public discourse about hospices: Cicely Saunders, who established St Christopher's Hospice in London, and Elisabeth Kübler-Ross, who rose to fame through publishing interviews with the terminally ill and introduced the once celebrated 'stage theory' of dying. A brief look at their biographies can serve to locate some early themes and trends in the development of the hospice movement and can also give some idea of the public appeal of that movement.

Some researchers have argued that the early British hospice movement could be classed as a charismatic movement, with Cicely Saunders as its charismatic leader (James and Field 1992). Saunders (1918–2005) fit well into British upper-middle class and upper-class models of 'charitable work' as a lifetime's calling; in fact, she was knighted in recognition of her achievements. After studying at Oxford, she was initially trained as a nurse, then as a charitable social worker, and later studied to be a doctor with the explicit aim of providing better care for the terminally ill. Saunders, who suffered from chronic back pain herself, became a prominent researcher and a pioneer in the medical treatment of pain during the 1960s and 1970s. She did her research, amongst other places, at St Christopher's Hospice, London, the world's first modern hospice, which she had founded in 1967. St Christopher's remains an international centre of the hospice movement to the present day. After a profound conversion experience in 1940, Saunders became and remained a devout Christian. In keeping with her initial training as a nurse and social worker, she put great emphasis on holistic care for all aspects of the person of the patient and for his family, but themes such as fighting death denial or staging opposition to the biomedical system, which are sometimes associated with the hospice movement, were not issues on her agenda.[13]

Elisabeth Kübler-Ross, the second figurehead of the hospice movement, took a somewhat different angle on things. She was born in Switzerland in 1926, moved to the U.S. in 1958, trained as a physician and became a psychiatrist. In the probably most popular book on death and dying ever (Kübler-Ross 1969), she developed a stage theory of dying, which has been very popular in some hospice circles, but is now viewed with some caution.[14]

Kübler-Ross's books about death and dying became world-wide bestsellers for many years, were translated into twenty-six languages and made her an international celebrity in the self-help, personal-growth market. She started a franchise system in the U.S. where one can train to be a certified counsellor in her system of ideas. While Cicely Saunders's spiritual inclination remained Christian, Elisabeth Kübler-Ross developed more innovative leanings early on and in the 1970s started to interpret dealing with death mainly as a chance for personal growth. She later proclaimed more and more esoteric viewpoints, with a bent towards spiritism and shamanism.

Elisabeth Kübler-Ross died in 2004. She was certainly not a biomedical positivist, and many of her publications are mostly aimed at audiences with an interest in new perspectives on life, personal growth and spirituality. Awareness of death was an important topic for her, and indeed it sometimes seems that for her and her audiences, contemplating death and the dying is predominantly a tool for self-development. Kübler-Ross's style and approach thus differ clearly from the more sober outlook of Cicely Saunders, but both can be taken to represent important currents within the hospice movement.

In the Anglophone world, hospices soon became widespread and partially integrated in the health system.[15] In Germany, however, the hospice movement caught on later. The introduction of hospices initially met with strong resistance, mainly from physicians who feared an isolation of dying patients from the rest of the health system. They were probably also concerned with a loss of status and reputation for their profession once the claims of the hospice proponents regarding its shortcomings were accepted as true. In his description of a Recklinghausen hospice, the first of its kind in Germany, Kirschner (1996: 51–52) gives details of the debate, which calmed down in the nineties but lingers on in attempts to integrate hospice services into larger hospital structures. In spite of it, first model institutions were opened in Cologne, Aachen and Recklinghausen in the early and mid-1980s, and by the mid-1990s there was a whole wave of hospices being founded all over Germany.[16]

The term 'hospice movement', suggesting an organised and goal-oriented impetus, can be misleading for the German context. In Germany, hospices were started independently from each other in different places, with different emphases and outlooks on their practice and sometimes looking directly to specific partner institutions in the U.K. or the U.S. for guidance. They did not manage to organise effective national structures until the mid-1990s. Those overarching organisations that now exist are still divided into several currents at the time of writing, the most visible organisations being the Bundesarbeitsgemeinschaft Hospiz (BAG), representing the actual hospice institutions, and the Deutsche Hospizstiftung, a private charity. The hospice movement is best seen as a grassroots, middle-class-based 'New Social Movement', rather than a centralised organisation with a coherent structure and ideology, and it is not always easy to generalise hospice ideology beyond the broader statements that have already been made concerning the Anglo-American roots of the hospice idea.

Pfeffer (1998: 33–34, 36) suggests that there are definite criteria typical of the German hospice movement on the whole which have to be met for a patient to be admitted to a hospice, such as conscious choice and awareness, acceptance of hospice principles, and rejection of certain types of medical treatment such as artificial feeding. In my own experience, while the fulfilment of these criteria was certainly an important goal at Stadtwald Hospice, they were not necessarily compulsory for patients to be admitted.

Palliative care units in hospitals have existed in Germany for almost as long as hospices, but were fewer in number. Such units are attached to hospitals like other specialised wards, such as oncology, gynaecology, or the like. While they focus on alleviating symptoms in much the same way as hospices do, they are organised in principle along standard biomedical lines. Unlike hospices, where patients are allowed to stay until the end of their lives if necessary, palliative wards in Germany aim at getting symptoms such as pain under control and send patients home, or back to an oncology ward, once this has been achieved. Their aims are thus not curative in a strict sense but still therapeutic by biomedical definitions. The medical speciality 'palliative medicine', which in Germany developed in the 1990s, can thus be interpreted as an attempt by mainstream biomedicine to reclaim territory lost to the hospice movement. While nurses, priests, psychotherapists and other professional groups play a large role and have prominent positions in the German hospice movement, palliative medicine is more exclusively dominated by physicians.[17]

Death, Denial and the Social Sciences

Having sketched the early history of the hospice movement as well as its social and discursive preconditions, it remains to be asked what role social scientists played in these developments taking place in their own societies. My claim is that there are intimate, if not always directly obvious, relations between the hospice idea, hospice practice and the social sciences.[18]

Most importantly, beginning in the late 1950s, social scientists were prominent in propagating the denial-of-death thesis, which has already been mentioned and which was to become an important intellectual context for the hospice movement. Almost a decade before the hospice movement was initiated, work by sociologists Geoffrey Gorer (1955, 1965), Herman Feifel (1959) and Peter L. Berger (Berger and Lieban 1960) started to portray Western industrial societies as denying death, which was to become a very popular charge in the following decades. Glaser and Strauss (1965a, 1968), in their groundbreaking work on medical sociology, also provided a context for the denial thesis – 'awareness' of death and dying, which they researched, became a major issue in public discourse.

With Peter L. Berger's and Thomas Luckmann's classic foundation texts on social constructionism (Berger and Luckmann 1966, Berger 1990[1967]), the denial thesis made it into sociological theory: culture, it was argued, is itself essentially a form of death denial, since death is the ultimate threat to ontological security. 'Every human society is, in the last resort, men banded together in the face of death' (Berger 1990[1967]: 51). The emphasis here is of course different, as all culture is concerned, and not specific types of Western societies, but the basic idea is quite similar.[19]

Central to the ensuing discussion about awareness and denial, which was soon taken up by non-academic writers, was the claim that death had been made a taboo and had been removed from public visibility in industrialised societies, while at the same time the dignity and individuality of dying patients were neglected by an overly hierarchical and technical biomedical system, and burials commercialised by the funeral industry (Mitford 1963). Such accusations were often combined with a general critique of positivist modernism and an inhumane biomedical system (Illich 1983[1976]). Frequently, historical (Ariès 1997[1978]) or anecdotal anthropological arguments for a 'better' or 'more natural' death were advanced to back up this view. Despite a few calls for caution (Fuchs 1971, Kellehear 1984), the denial-of-death thesis was the main position in the media and social sciences in Germany and elsewhere in the 1970s and 1980s and was often proposed with great zeal. It also came to dominate public opinion almost completely to the present day, an interesting contradiction in itself.[20]

One author of an early bibliography on death, dying and bereavement pointed out that it was odd how more than 650 titles about an allegedly taboo topic could be in print and publicly available (Simpson 1987[1979]: vii). Some writers have still argued in favour of the denial thesis (Elias 1985, Nassehi and Weber 1989),

11

while others, more recently, reject it straight away (Feldmann 1997, Seale 1998). The most convincing position at present seems that adopted by Walter (1991, 1994) and Mellor (1993), who point out that there is no evidence to back up the claim that death is a taboo topic. However, rather than dismissing the denial thesis altogether, they suggest that attention needs to be paid to the question as to which representations of death and which death-related practices in which segments of society are being discussed. Following a theoretical framework developed by Giddens (1991), Mellor argues that death today is sequestrated into the private realm by reflexive individualising tendencies of high modernity, and hospice institutions ultimately support this tendency (Mellor 1993: esp. 18–21). Such more recent positions are typical for contemporary approaches to death denial in that they differentiate the meanings of the term 'denial' and the social contexts in question so finely that the initial pro and contra positions have now largely lost their meaning.

However, outside the academic realm, denial-of-death and vague allegations of insufficient treatment of dying patients by society in general and biomedical institutions in particular continue to be important arguments in favour of hospices to this day. Even where such arguments are historicised as a phenomenon from the past, they still serve as a kind of founding myth. Regardless of its truth content, this rhetoric enabled the hospice movement to back its general goals with a precise and compelling moral appeal. It also helped to portray the hospice idea as being distinct from mainstream biomedicine and morally superior to it, a claim which overemphasises the actual blurred boundaries between the two approaches, and their internal inconsistencies.

The denial thesis also enabled social scientists to follow their professional calling and bring to light an aspect of the social, namely death and dying, purportedly hitherto concealed from the public eye. Clive Seale (1998: 139–40) points out that there is an epistemological connection between patient-centred medicine and qualitative research in their shared emphasis on the validity of individual experience over the truth claims of more abstract systems of knowledge and power. David Armstrong (1987: 656), in his Foucauldian critique of Philippe Ariès (1997[1978]), characterises those social scientists who detected and fought 'death denial' as self-appointed humanists, who see themselves as solving a mystery and liberating death, while failing to recognise that they are part of the same discourse they purport to examine.

From today's point of view, charges of death denial, spelled out by social scientists, had an important legitimating function for all those professionals – nurses, doctors, therapists and researchers – who were to make a living in the new field of discourse and practice which 'dying' was to become. Social scientists, then, should not only ask why death and dying as topics were overlooked but also why such topics came up and were created at all and what role their disciplines played in such a process. On a more personal level, this is the question I will pursue in the next chapter, with regard to myself as a researcher.

Notes

1. For the sake of clarity, I shall quote Fernandez (1986), which is a collection of essays published at earlier dates, as if it were a monograph. The same is true for the later notation Geertz (1995[1973]), which really refers to the German translation of an English compilation of earlier essays.

2. The title of a popular nursing textbook for the subject, which went through several editions and is called *Sterbebeistand, Sterbebegleitung, Sterbegeleit*, is indicative here (Rest 1998[1989]). An English translation is difficult, approximately: 'support in dying, company in dying, escort in dying'.

3. I owe the idea of treating 'dying' as a field of thought and practice emerging in the context of a quite recent discourse to Arnar Arnason (1998), who draws on the work of Michel Foucault in his study of bereavement counselling. One alternative introduction to the anthropology of death 'at home' can be found in Salis Gross' study of death in a Swiss home for the elderly (2001: 25–63): it is organised around the three dominant contemporary images of denied death, terrifying death and natural death. My own account in the remainder of this chapter is by no means meant to compete with detailed historical or sociological analyses; my aim is rather to outline and clarify concepts and developments needed for the later ethnographic chapters.

4. While I use the term biomedicine in a generalising fashion throughout this text for clarity's sake, it is not my intention to claim that biomedicine is a unified, coherent field of discourse and practice – of course it has its own contradictions and inconsistencies, which need not be discussed in detail here. For one definition of the biomedical model of illness, see Armstrong (2000: 25), who also sketches the history of the involvement of the social sciences with medicine.

5. Not all patients at Stadtwald hospice were clearly 'informed' of their terminal prognosis, an issue I shall return to later.

6. Anthropological and sociological analyses in this context are, amongst others, Lock (2000) and, for the German context, Lindemann (2002) and Schneider (1999a, 1999b). Views from several disciplines are collected in Schlich and Wiesemann (2001).

7. My own translation, emphasis in the original.

8. There are several vantage points from which social theorists describe the processes in question. Rose (1989) follows Michel Foucault and analyses power effects in the formation of the reflexive self. Giddens (1991), prefers to write of reflexive modernisation, and its ever increasing feedback loops. Mellor and Shilling (1993) extend Giddens' theoretical framework to the analysis of death and dying. Bauman (1992) stresses postmodern aspects of self-formation and its relation to death. I found all three points of view useful as analytical tools for my ethnographic work.

9. Of course, there is an ideological assumption of personhood and of the individual here, the term of ownership is not coincidental, and I shall analyse this further in my ethnographic chapters. The coinage 'one's own death' is taken from Walter (1994).

10. The term 'social death' was originally coined by Glaser and Strauss (1965a, 1968) and also used in Sudnow's ethnographic study (1967). According to these authors, people are socially dead when they are treated in their presence as if they were not there. This definition is based on Goffman's (1959) notion of the non-person. Macho (1987) was, to my knowledge, the first writer to argue that any death is primarily a social death. For earlier discussions of social death see also Mulkay (1993) and Weber (1994); for a survey of the changing approaches to social death in the social sciences see Mulkay and Ernst (1991).

11. Lawton (2000: 122–47) sees the sequestration of unbounded bodies as an additional important social function of hospices, and discusses that point in detail. Probably because of the specifics of my own fieldwork context, this was not an issue that seemed equally striking to me at Stadt-

wald hospice. Still, Lawton's observation fits extremely well with the ideologies of self and biography that I observed in my own fieldwork.

12. See Kirschner (1996: 48–57) and, for a historical survey of hospice issues in the German press since the 1970s, Seitz and Seitz (2002). For a comparative view of the situation of hospice care in Europe see Gronemeyer et al. (2004).

13. Clark (2002) has edited a large number of Saunders's letters and gives brief introductions to different phases of her life. The popular biography by DuBoulay (1987) also provides a list of her earlier publications (DuBoulay 1987: 220–22).

14. It is argued by some that the stage theory is too general, too prescriptive, and mainly appeals to those with little first-hand exposure to death and dying (Howe 1992: 54–68). The German version of *On Death and Dying* (Kübler-Ross 1969) is *Interviews mit Sterbenden* (1987[1971]). A very sympathetic account of the work of Kübler-Ross is given by Gantois Chaban (2000). Kübler-Ross's early life before 1969 is recounted by Gill (1984[1981]). For her ideas, an impression of her work and a full list of her publications see also www.elisabethkublerross.com.

15. In fact, they became subject to large-scale scientific surveys in the 1980s (Greer and Mor 1986, Greer et al. 1986, Seale 1989, Johnson et al. 1990).

16. At the time of my research, hospice foundation in Germany was so rapid that the figures available had been overtaken by developments by the time they appeared, and there is now academic research activity concerning hospice care in Germany comparable to that in Britain in the 1990s. An overview of statistical details, addresses etc. is Sabatowski (1999 and yearly later editions). Clark (1991) mentions similar initial resistance to hospices in Britain.

17. See, for example, Pichlmaier (1998), Aulbert and Zech (1997) and Klaschik (2000) for German palliative medicine, and Müller and Kern (2002) for a short comparison of hospices and palliative wards in Germany.

18. My reading of British sociology of death and dying, notably Walter (1993, 1994), Mellor and Shilling (1993) and Seale (1998), prompted me to think about the involvement – or lack thereof – of the social sciences in the study of death. A discussion of the role of the discipline of sociology from the German perspective is found in Feldmann and Fuchs-Heinritz (1995a), who, however, avoid any self-reflexive considerations. By 'social sciences' I generally mean all those scientific disciplines concerned with the social, namely social or cultural anthropology, sociology, German 'Europäische Ethnologie', cultural studies and social psychology.

19. Anthony Giddens (1991) also uses this argument. Ultimately, I believe this position is a 'culturalisation' of Heidegger's (2001[1927]) thanatology (see Ebeling 1979b). From an ethnographic perspective, I suspect that death is the ultimate and paramount test case of ontological security, as passionately argued by Peter L. Berger (1990[1967]), mainly for intellectuals.

20. One good, recent summary of the debates about a denial of death can be found in Salis Gross (2001: 27–44).

2
THE RESEARCH PROCESS

ೲೲ

Reflexivity and the Origins of the Ethnography

At the beginning of my ethnographic work, I was broadly interested in death, dying and the hospice movement in Germany. I started my research with the guiding assumption that the precise question and topic were to be specified as part of the research process. An interest, more a general direction than a clear topic, would thus be progressively differentiated, hoping to generate questions that were also part of the field and not exclusively proposed to it from the outside. As a result, the study took shape in a continuous dialectics between the initial topic, the field itself, and myself as a researcher. The field, the topic and the ethnographer in his mutually dependent roles as a researcher and an assistant nurse were constituted in the research process and shaped its further direction in turn.

Reflecting upon the vicissitudes of such a research process can in itself lead to important findings about the topic and place the results in context. In this sense, reflexivity and its written, to some degree necessarily personal, narration have become a general attitude in most of the discipline of anthropology. It is now largely the individual ethnographer's choice to decide on which aspects of his research and writing he deems giving a reflexive account necessary and appropriate.[1]

There are three main aspects I want to emphasise with regard to my own position: First, I intend to use a degree of reflexivity to locate myself as a researcher. Pierre Bourdieu (1999[1993]), for example, argues that reflexivity in the social sciences should primarily, or even exclusively, be used to outline the social conditions of the production of the producer of knowledge. Understood in this way, reflexivity tries to locate the researcher and his scientific interests within the common practices of larger social groups, including the academic field.

Second, I intend to use reflexive writing in order to put the reader in a position to understand and critically evaluate constitutive steps in the research process. She should be enabled, at least to some degree, to judge how I positioned myself as an ethnographer towards the research topic, and to understand how my field was delineated and thereby created. This is important not so much for judging the objectivity of the results, but for elucidating their nature as specifically situated – not absolute or objective – knowledge.

My third and final intention is to employ reflexivity in order to learn from the initial strangeness that my entry into my field engendered, and from spontaneous personal reactions I had towards fieldwork and towards the experiences during fieldwork when I wrote my diaries. As will become apparent in the ethnographic chapters, my participant observation often took place under conditions of hard physical labour, I frequently lacked time and was sometimes emotionally exposed. This left traces of a personal nature in my diary writing and in my analysis of hospice life. I shall occasionally depart from Bourdieu's admonition and reflect upon these traces.[2]

I began working on this study late in 1998 when I moved to Berlin with the aim of conducting participatory research in anthropology about the hospice movement. I was expecting that this would place my work in the field of the anthropology of religion and that the focus of my fieldwork would be on how hospice patients thought about their own approaching death. Abstract meaning-making in the face of death was a central interest of mine and I expected such meaning-making to make use of predominantly religious, psychotherapeutic and philosophical concepts. From a more theoretical point of view, I expected to describe and analyse symbolic cultural systems through 'thick description', as advocated by Clifford Geertz (1995[1973]). This was going to be my first ethnographic research project, and I was very interested in participant observation as a method, not least because it was to give me a break from the study of written historical documents.

As a researcher, I was thus part of the discourse on death, dying and hospice work outlined above: an academically trained person with an upper-middle class background, who hoped to make some personal philosophical headway by reflexively engaging with death through the methodology of an *en vogue* subject, cultural anthropology. Significantly, this was not my first contact with the hospice movement. As an undergraduate, I had for a short time worked as a volunteer in a hospice group. I was therefore part of the wider social field already and only changed sides to the academic shore.[3]

In a six-week Red Cross training course, I acquired some basic nursing skills that would prove useful in my fieldwork. During the practical part of the course, I worked for two weeks in a nursing home for the elderly. This gave me a first idea of what nursing could be like under less than ideal circumstances in an understaffed and under-funded health care institution. After a year of reading, training, grant applications and other preparatory work, I introduced myself to several hospice managers and had preliminary talks about conducting my research in their institutions. After a number of such talks the manager of one hospice in a northern German city agreed that I could work there, initially as an intern in nursing. At approximately the same time, I received a research grant and could thus dedicate myself fully to fieldwork.

Background Information about Stadtwald Hospice

Not surprising for grass-roots institutions which proclaim a liberal, choice-oriented ideology, German hospices show diverse characteristics in their setting, their funding, their routines, their approaches to nursing care and their atmosphere. They make a point of this, too. Some are Christian, others are secular, some are situated in representative nineteenth century houses, others in modern high-rises. Quite a few are managed by priests, others by doctors, psychologists or nurses. The number of patient beds available is normally somewhere between five and twenty.

Stadtwald Hospice, where I worked, was a relatively recently founded institution, situated in a working-class area of a northern German city. The initiative for the foundation had come from two oncology nurses, who had felt that circumstances in their ward were insufficient to provide adequate terminal care. When they decided to get together and start planning a project for terminal care, they had not heard of the hospice idea and the hospice movement yet, but immediately liked the concept when they came across it. They gathered a group of volunteers, mostly from nursing professions, and worked towards their project for several years in their spare time, without pay and overcoming considerable organisational challenges.[4]

When they finally managed to secure adequate funding, at least temporarily, they went ahead and founded a charitable company of which they became the managers. The hospice began its work with the admission of the first patient, and some of the volunteers from the founding group started to work there full time. One of the managers left later, after disagreements which were partly of a personal nature, and partly due to the administrative changes between the improvisation of the founding period and the more routine later management requirements.[5] From the beginning, the hospice did not have any religious ties or explicit agenda to this effect, which made it interesting for my research, as I initially hoped to work with patients of different religious denominations in a neutral setting.

The twenty-eight people who were employed full time by the hospice when I first worked there were mostly women, but the percentage of men was to rise sharply in the following years. There were twenty nurses, the manager, a social worker, three administrative staff, a cook, some kitchen staff and cleaning staff.

Quite a number of people worked part time, and the music therapist, supervising staff psychotherapists and some nurses worked on a freelance basis. Depending on doctors' prescriptions, specialised doctors and members of other health professions would come in from the outside. Finally, there were about fifty unpaid volunteers – at least on the volunteer list – working in nursing, in the kitchen, in administration or in bereavement groups. Their involvement ranged from an infrequent couple of hours to one or two days per week. In actual fact, I encountered very few volunteers in nursing-related work areas at Stadtwald Hospice, the exception being kitchen staff.

The hospice had fifteen beds, and 139 patients stayed there during the year my fieldwork began, with similar figures in the following years. Almost all of them died in the hospice. Most patients came from financially modest backgrounds, and there were only a few university graduates amongst them. Frequent professions were sales, housekeeping, clerical work and construction. Sixty percent of patients were women, and the average age of patients was sixty-four. However, there were extreme deviations from this. One patient I met was twenty-five, another ninety-four. A patient's stay in the hospice averaged thirty-two days, but again there were large deviations from that value. Almost all patients had cancer, and cancers of the brain, the lungs and the otorhinolaryngal tracts were the most frequent. There were hardly any patients with HIV, mainly since a number of institutions specialising in HIV care already existed and also because of rapid progress in HIV treatment at the time of my research. It shall be the task of later chapters of this study to introduce some of the patients I met and individualise the impersonal data given here.[6]

In the hospice, I received the following account of the relation between hospice, nursing homes and hospitals: hospitals, including palliative wards, had strictly defined missions, always aiming at healing or at least at a significant improvement of a patient's condition. This was prescribed by arrangements with insurance companies and was in accordance with the curative ideal of biomedicine. Therefore, hospitals had no interest in keeping those patients for whom there was no chance for cure or lasting improvement, and there were also no financial provisions for such patients by insurance companies. Both were thus interested in sending terminally ill patients back to their own homes, which was the cheapest option, or to nursing homes. Nursing homes in turn were normally not interested at all in admitting such patients, as they were likely to consume a lot of already scarce resources and were unlikely to stay for long because of their terminal prognosis. At home, however, relatives were often stretched to the limit of what they could cope with by looking after cancer patients. This again could result in patients being repeatedly sent back to hospital through emergency services by their helpless relatives. So while everybody involved agreed in principle that it was best to let patients die at home, still a cycle of back and forth movement between private home and health care institutions could ensue. This was very hard for patients, often already totally exhausted by their illness and taxing years of strenuous therapies. Admission to a hospice could serve, in principle, as a way out.[7]

The most important criterion for admission was that, for whatever reason, a patient could not be looked after at home by relatives or mobile nursing services, while, at the same time, there was no further indication for curative treatment. Many patients who came to Stadtwald Hospice were relieved to be able to stay in one place and be looked after without having to worry about their relatives or the next impending change of location. Admission could be from home or from a hospital, but not from a nursing home. This rule aimed at preventing nursing homes from offloading work or cost-intensive patients onto the hospice. At the time of my fieldwork, there was a forty-to-seventy person waiting list for admission, but not everybody on the list needed a place straight away.

The hospice cooperated closely with mobile doctors' teams who specialised in the care of cancer patients at home. These doctors continued to look after patients once they were admitted, and financial and administrative matters were organised as if doctors were to visit patients at home. Since these doctors had often known patients for quite some time before they applied for admission to the hospice, their judgement weighed quite heavily with the hospice social worker who assessed individual applications. Another important channel for admission to the hospice was that of hospital social workers, who often introduced patients and their relatives to the hospice idea, helped to establish initial personal contacts and sometimes already put patients on the hospice waiting list.

Hospice costs differed from patient to patient, but were cheaper than hospital costs in most cases. The exact total amount billed to the insurance agencies depended on the individual bills for medication and specialist treatment, which were billed separately from hospice running costs. In 1999, the year before I started my research, daily running costs per patient were 520 DM. The hospice had to provide 10 percent of these running costs through donations or voluntary work. About 350 DM were provided for by insurance agencies, and 50 DM by patients, their families or welfare agencies. The remainder of all expenditures was paid for by the federal state in which Stadtwald Hospice was situated.

The Emergence of Field, Topic and Researcher

Being a model institution and one of the first of its kind in the region, Stadtwald Hospice attracted a lot of attention right from the start. While I was doing my own research, visits from journalists and local television teams were not infrequent. Medical interns worked in nursing for some time out of personal interest, a psychotherapist worked on her M.A. thesis, and shortly after my own fieldwork was completed, another social scientist started to do research there. Guided tours for groups of visitors were a standard routine for the hospice manager and administrative staff.

The hospice also looked for publicity quite actively as part of its fundraising efforts. Many staff were used to dealing with journalists and cameras. One member of the nursing team once told me that she should not smile into the camera as this showed the wrinkles on her face. This demonstrates that she had seen herself on television and was not only expecting to appear there again, but also to shape impressions actively. At another time, a request for a visit from a television team was declined because, as a nurse said on the phone, the hospice was being renovated and thus did not make for very good pictures at the time. The management of publicity and information through personal conduct when meeting journalists, through publishing brochures and through organising fundraising events was thus approached in quite an aware and professional way.

Additionally, the model character of the hospice had made a period of training there part of the curriculum for a number of health professions: student nurses came for modules of their course, high school students for professional orientation week, university students of psychology and medicine for voluntary internships, and nurses for the elderly did their professional recognition internship at the hospice. Some of the freelance nurses working at the hospice were studying at university for higher vocational degrees in nursing management or nursing training. The hospice manager was often invited to give talks outside. Thus, the hospice was very closely connected to all sorts of educational institutions, and many people from such institutions spent some time of their training there.

Because of the attention by the media and the presence of so many people in their training, the coming and going of people with different motivations, different backgrounds and different qualifications was part of the everyday working life of the full-time nurses. For them, there was always a new face to get used to, some nosy question to be answered, somebody to whom some nursing task needed to be explained. Many of these temporary visitors would, however, also lend a welcome hand to the senior nurses or provide more publicity. Additionally, there was the expected coming and going of patients. In all, Stadtwald Hospice had an institutional atmosphere which easily accommodated fluctuation. Even of the full-time staff itself, about one-quarter left in the three years during which I was in close contact with the hospice – still a comparatively low turnover for a German nursing institution, as I was told.

The welcoming atmosphere in the hospice, which made the start of my fieldwork much easier, was of course not simply disinterested generosity. Behind it lay the desire to spread hospice ideals, and in fact the hospice management hoped to gain a little feedback and publicity from my work.

Once I had started to work as an assistant nurse, I was surprised to find that self-reflexive, qualitative research approaches and participatory methods were very well received by staff. I soon realised that reflexivity was part of the daily work of hospice nurses; if they did not already have a propensity to do so, they were prompted through supervision sessions to think about their nursing practice and their reasons for working at a hospice for dying patients. On a less conscious, but all the more significant plane, nurses were engaged in discussions about the behaviour of patients, about communication with patients and about their own role in it, on a daily basis. For anyone working at the hospice, the confrontation with the biographical, psychological and social situation of patients made it a very small step indeed to questioning one's own life projects and points of view. In fact, many nurses had chosen to work at the hospice because they wanted to work in an environment that allowed and encouraged such reflexivity. As a result of this approach to their work, and of many years of experience, many of the full-time staff were very skilled in the identification and management of emotions, including quite veiled or subconscious ones, in themselves and others. They were as good in the professional use of emotional disclosure as in the authoritative drawing of boundaries.

They were also used to dealing with much more disruptive feelings and situations than those an initially very timid participant observer could have caused. In retrospect, I find my anthropologist's conviction that I could potentially cause a lot of disruption in my chosen field a little amusing – from the point of view of the conscious management of emotions and social relations, my 'field' was far more professional and aware than I was.

Thus, Stadtwald Hospice had a specific institutional atmosphere which was generally conducive for starting my fieldwork as a participant observer and assistant nurse. Within that atmosphere, it became my task to negotiate a position in which I could gain some insight into hospice nursing and conduct my research in a productive manner. Such negotiation remained an ongoing process during my fieldwork as an assistant nurse/participant observer, which took place over a period of two years and consisted of three phases of approximately two months each. In every one of these phases, my role was different, giving me different perspectives on Stadtwald Hospice. In turn, different perspectives prompted me to revise my idea of the hospice and caused me to redirect my research. Because I had a very active role in all of this, rather than discovering or investigating my field, I would prefer to speak of constructing it.[8]

The most important logistical balance I needed to strike was between exposure to nursing practice on the one hand and workload on the other. During the first part of my fieldwork I worked full shifts like all nurses, five days a week, approximately thirty days in total. After every shift, I sat down for several hours to write my diaries. This led to an extremely demanding work routine, but gave me good exposure to hospice nursing and resulted in very useful diary accounts. My colleagues accepted my presence without problems, and the working consensus seemed to be that I would be well accepted as long as I worked full shifts and did not cause any major interruptions in nursing routines. Thus, my research had a good start, but it did not seem possible to take notes during my actual work, to use tape recorders or to drop out of my nursing role in order to continue an interesting conversation with a patient, or the like. I was more of a recollecting participant than a participant observer – not necessarily a disadvantage, as this allowed me to submerge myself fully in nursing work without withdrawing continually from the action.

However, during my second research period, I tried to stress my role as a researcher over my role as a nurse and to find an arrangement that was less physically exhausting. I worked fewer days and tried to have days off for diary writing between shifts. I mentioned my research much more often to patients and offered presentations of preliminary results to members of staff, which, however, were quite poorly attended. I also tried to widen the scope of my work by conducting interviews with nurses and following up research threads outside the hospice, such as talking to a hospice psychotherapist and accompanying a cancer doctor on his daily round through town.

By this time, I was very well integrated in the hospice and quite friendly with many of my colleagues, who considered me a reliable work partner within the limits of my qualifications. I enjoyed working there, I had gained enough experience to be much more relaxed at work and I understood patients and daily nursing practice much better than before. The diaries of that period were fewer, but more detailed. However, the fact that I worked only intermittently gave me the feeling that I missed out on a lot of decisive developments in the care of individual patients, so I changed my approach again for the last research period.

In that last period, I was taken off the staff rota and thus free to withdraw to write my diaries after a couple of hours' work in one shift. In this way, I managed to write my most detailed texts without being overworked and yet with a continuous presence in the hospice. This time, however, since staff could not rely on counting me in for the daily schedule, I was only given tasks of secondary importance and felt I was somewhat left on the sidelines of nursing practice.

I concluded that the dilemma between a field with intensive work demands and high work ethics in nursing, on the one hand, and the researcher's interest in both continuous exposure and space for writing, on the other, could simply not be resolved. It was itself a defining feature of my field and my participant observation. By coincidence, rather than by planning, it turned out that I emphasised specific aspects of that dilemma during different research periods, which provided me not with an ideal solution, but with an overall well rounded insight within the above limitations.

These were not the only limitations. Another specific set of conditions for my research was imposed by my social role as an assistant nurse. My perspective was not identical to that of the fully qualified nurses. Even leaving aside the obvious fact that a researcher remains primarily that a considerable amount of the time, a number of more practical limitations applied: I was, for example, not admitted to the weekly staff meeting, in which full-time nurses and management discussed problems of the everyday running of the hospice, and, on a more practical plane, I had neither the training nor the permission to carry out many more advanced nursing tasks.

In relation to patients, a number of limitations applied as well: First of all, the fact that I was not a fully trained nurse meant that I was, in private and medical matters, only a secondary partner for patients, who tended to discuss important issues with those having higher qualifications, more experience and authority. Indeed, I had to refer patients to other nurses for many such matters. Also, while the temporary insight into patients' lives was very direct and intimate, the fact that patients were alone during most of the day must not be overlooked – my insight into most of their lives at the hospice remained, of course, limited to the time of nursing interaction.

As may already have become apparent, I now think that my approach was initially quite timid. I was eager to be accepted, very careful not to cause any disruptions, preoccupied with fears of being intrusive and of my research failing right from the start. While I could probably have made faster progress from the point of view of social science data gathering, from the ethnographic point of view, the fact that I was willing to take time, invest effort, and be self-critical was well received and ultimately proved quite productive.

In all, my position in the hospice was very specific, situated in a web of social interactions and relationships, inseparable from my own physical presence, my personality and my social roles as assistant nurse and ethnographer. It is best described, in the words of Aaron Turner (2000), as a 'socially constitutive configuration', which is neither 'from their point of view' nor 'distorted by the ethnographers' presence'. My understanding of my role as an ethnographer is not that I speak as an initiated insider of a uniform hospice culture, nor that I present the complete ethnography of an 'institution'. Neither am I a detached 'observer', though. Rather, I write from a specific social position that loses no validity by being personal, interactive and changing.[9]

From the point of view of patient-centred nursing, May states what is equally true for the participant observer in a nursing role: 'It is important to note that the 'knowledge' about patients on which individualised care depends is always provisional and never complete: the discontinuity of nurse-patient relationships, the clinical trajectory of the patient, and a number of other factors – notably the extent to which the patient is willing to talk about her or himself – will inhibit its collection and collation.' (May 1993: 1365) I may add that this is, for both the nurse and the participant observer, a matter of course and ultimately quite all right.

The process of negotiating a research role and realising its scope and limitations was paralleled by a continuous development of my idea of the topic and direction of my work. Not unexpectedly, ideas about what exactly it was that I was looking for changed with the construction of the field I worked in and with my changing understanding of it. Reflexive methodology enabled me to make productive use of the changes that such a process caused in my agenda, to learn from them and gain insights about my topic, rather than see them as a shameful distortion of an initial research design.

In the beginning, I had considered the hospice a place in which patients, nurses and relatives, through the implementation of hospice ideals, dealt with a central aspect of their existence, namely death and mortality. I wanted to find out how hospice practice was constituted in the interaction of those groups, and how meaning was found in this situation. While this quite general scope remained the same, entering the field and becoming acquainted with it changed my understanding of what my research was about in at least three important ways. The first change was from a focus on death to a focus on life. As staff had predicted to me early on, I soon realised that death would remain an inaccessible category not only with respect to philosophical theory, but also in social practice. My research turned out to be primarily about severe illness and about nursing, and by all means about life. I had to part from my initial implicit assumption that dying revealed something about death – at least not in the way that I had expected.

In close connection with the above-mentioned shift, my attention turned from the abstract, discursive involvement with death, which I had expected from patients and staff, to everyday practices, routines of nursing and daily projects and problems of patients. I realised that my own academic background, parts of the academic literature and the presentation of the hospice movement in the media had provided me with the mistaken stereotype that death and dying prompted abstract ethical and philosophical considerations in patients and staff. The search for meaning, I learned, was most prominent in seemingly banal, often non-discursive everyday practices, not in the discussion of grand ideas.

Finally, my theoretical attention shifted from the description of symbolic systems in Geertz's sense (1995[1973]) to the analysis of narrative. I soon found a conceptualisation of culture as a symbolic system inadequate when it came to describing the decisive aspects of hospice life and my own position within them. I found no more or less uniform 'hospice culture', but became involved in patterns of social interaction and everyday nursing practice in which I was an active participant myself. The challenge was to analyse the ways in which these patterns were structured and perpetuated. Narrative theory turned out to be especially well suited for doing so.

The above-mentioned changes in the research process can be metaphorically described as a movement from the outside to the inside, as a crossing of two boundaries: the boundary between theoretical anthropology as intellectual activity and concrete participation in fieldwork, and the boundary between the outside representation and the inside practice of the hospice. In the present case, these boundaries largely coincided. In the process of crossing them, categories which were important on the outside – such as death, medicine, symbols, consciousness, ethical problems or abstract talk, to name only the most important – were replaced by their equivalents from the inside perspective, and I came to see the at times surprising other side of the coin. Death became superseded by life, medicine by nursing, symbols by stories, consciousness by ambivalence, ethical problems by emotional pragmatism, abstract talk by metaphor.

24

A Note on Research Ethics, Diaries and Translations

Initially, I had been somewhat shy to mention my research to patients, and at the same time I felt that it was extremely important that they knew exactly what I was doing. With time, I managed to bring the topic up with quite a number of patients. In those cases where that seemed feasible, I tried to introduce my research method and agenda, and to discuss the involvement of patients and their lives in it, but I hardly ever met with much interest, be it approval or rejection. Characteristically, there would be a short, somewhat positive reaction which may have been just politeness ('Oh, yes, the State University, interesting...'), but no further interest to learn anything more. In addition, many patients were simply not able to have longer conversations with me and spent their remaining energy on more immediate concerns.

More importantly, however, the question as to whether patients were 'informed' about their prognosis and 'knew' about impending death and what the hospice was about, proved tricky and ambiguous. From the point of view of doctors and staff, some patients were fully informed; others were not yet but would be soon. In most cases, however, while there had been very frank conversations and no information was concealed, it could not automatically be assumed that patients were conscious of all they had been told all the time, or wanted to be confronted with it again. In the course of my research, 'awareness' and 'being informed', both key aspects of patient-centred medicine, medical ethics and the hospice movement, increasingly appeared to me as categories which only very inaccurately described the patients' state of information and consciousness, and their changing conceptualisations of their illness. Awareness seemed to be a possibly very temporary phenomenon, interpreted differently by different social actors, in different relationships and at different times.[10]

Apart from the patients' frequent lack of interest and energy, I did not want to force information on people who, temporarily or permanently, had chosen not to deal with the issue of death. In such cases, I tried to use phrases such as 'I study hospices...' or 'I am interested in severe illness and death...'. However, for all the above reasons, I hardly ever managed to solicit an explicit, textbook style informed consent from a patient, not so much for lack of consent but for disinterest in information.[11]

Hospice staff saw no problem in this and found my concerns odd when I repeatedly insisted on it being problematic. They knew that I cared, and that seemed enough. Nurses at Stadtwald Hospice could be very protective of their patients. The concern as to what kind of anonymous information would come up about these patients in an ethnographic study for academic audiences was not one that made them feel protective at all. In the course of my research, I myself also attributed less and less importance to such issues – they receded without being resolved. By the end of my research, the question as to why I had approached the field with all sorts of preconceived abstract ideas about informed consent and purported dilemmas in research ethics seemed more interesting to me than the question as to how I solved or did not solve them.

I concluded that the expectation that I was engaging with an 'ethically problematic field' was suggested to me by media representations of death and dying on the one hand, and on the other hand by fellow researchers, mostly from the U.K. and the U.S., displaying the specific interpretations of research ethics prevalent in their training and academic culture. It is this expectation and the notion of 'informed consent' itself which should come under much closer ethnographic scrutiny in future studies.[12]

The issues of patients' awareness of their impending death and of patients' awareness of my research both had common roots in the liberal, self-reflexive and autonomous conception of the person discussed in chapter one. Severe illness frequently led to ambivalences and contradictions in both areas. As will be shown throughout this study, precisely this conception of the person is put in question by the circumstances of severe cancer. My failure to elicit informed consent is thus a rather typical phenomenon for the field I studied, and my initial concern with research ethics probably tells more about the social world I came from than about the one I entered.[13]

This is not to argue that no caution should be taken to protect the privacy of nurses and patients. During my research, I discussed questions of privacy with the hospice manager on a number of occasions. Wherever excerpts from my ethnographic diaries are used in the following chapters, patients' and nurses' names have been changed. In cases where the same name would have occurred frequently and in different passages, several different names were sometimes used. Where this seemed necessary in order to guarantee anonymity, elements of the description of patients, such as a rare kind of illness or a peculiar life history, have also been left out or were replaced by functionally similar accounts. The final text was given to the manager, to an English speaking nurse and to a supervising therapist from Stadtwald Hospice, to look over.

The indented texts appearing in the following chapters are excerpts from my fieldwork diaries which I have selected to illustrate specific points. The diaries were written down from memory as stream-of-consciousness type narratives at the end of each work shift, or directly after a talk or interview. Sometimes I also took very sketchy notes at handover and used these for my diaries. Writing usually took between one and three hours. I looked over the resulting texts a day or two later, reworked what was still incongruous, added some information from memory and then left the resulting text unchanged – except of course for the translation, which I did myself, and for some slight changes during the editing of the manuscript. Where the language of the diary excerpts has remained awkward or difficult to read, it is my responsibility, not the publisher's.

In translation, I tried not to straighten grammar and expressions when they were colloquial, sketchy or vague in the German original. I did not correct punctuation either. Where I was uncertain about the exact translation of a German term, I have left the original German expression in square brackets. Also appearing in square brackets are German technical terms from the field of nursing which seemed significant but could not easily be rendered in English, and explanatory text which I have inserted into the fieldwork diary excerpts in order to make them more intelligible for readers. In the following text, whenever someone is referred to by their first name without further explanation, they are fully employed nursing staff. Whenever someone is referred to as Mr or Mrs with their surnames, they are patients.

Notes

1. I see three main currents within anthropology and ethnographic writing from which a self-reflexive attitude stems. In actual practice, these often blend and are thus best described as ideal types. One position argues that a degree of reflexivity eliminates the subjectivity of the researcher to the greatest possible extent, and thus makes it possible to derive 'more objective facts' from qualitative methodology. This view is not so popular in anthropology today but is more widespread in sociology. Pierre Bourdieu's work, for example, points in this direction. A second root of reflexive methodology is feminist scholarship, with its emphasis on objectivity being a white, middle-class, male domain. One good example amongst many is Mascia-Lees et al. (1989); a corresponding epistemology is sketched by Haraway (1988). The third current in question is poststructuralism, which emphasises and analyses the ethnographer's position as a necessarily subjective author of texts and often celebrates the potential of ethnography as a personal, almost literary activity, e.g. most contributions to Clifford and Marcus (1986). This trend is summarised exhaustively, if somewhat uncritically, by Tedlock (1991) and more analytically by Berg and Fuchs (1999[1993]b). Waldenfels (1999: 117–51) presents a critical philosophical analysis of the discussions of representation and reflexivity in anthropology. He argues convincingly that, from a philosophical position, these problems are here to stay. See also Lindner (1981, 1988, 1995) for insightful positions on reflexivity and fieldwork.
2. This understanding of my self-reflexive position as an author and producer of knowledge is one point where my own approach differs from other studies on German hospices: Kirschner (1996), Pfeffer (1998) and Gerstenkorn (2004) mostly chose to remain invisible, either as actors or as narrators or both.
3. Again, Rest's (1998[1989]) textbook on death and dying for nursing students, encompassing and mixing discourses from nursing, spirituality, humanist psychotherapy, social sciences and poetry, can serve as a representative document of the atmosphere I experienced in a hospice group when trained as a hospice volunteer at the time.
4. The information in this and the following paragraphs stems mostly from talks with the hospice manager and the hospice social worker. The statistical information is that which was available at the time of my fieldwork, starting in 2000, published in a yearly hospice brochure. See also Kirschner (1996), Pfeffer (1998), Gerstenkorn (2004) and now Dreßke (2005) for comparative material from other German hospices. The German context described here is remarkably different from the situation of hospices abroad, e.g. those within the NHS in Britain. As will become apparent, Stadtwald Hospice had a physical structure, ethos and administrative framework which seem to make it quite a different institution from the hospices studied by Lawton (2000) and Hockey (1990).
5. James and Field (1992) have discussed the situation British hospices face when moving from an early, charismatic founding phase to later, more routine work. During my fieldwork, there were some signs that Stadtwald Hospice was undergoing a similar transformation.

6. Pfeffer's (1998: 41) group of patients falls in similar categories. In comparison to those at Stadtwald Hospice, the patients in the hospice she studied were, however, on average nine years older, less of them suffered from cancer (75 percent) and a higher percentage left the hospice again (30 percent), which was a very rare exception at Stadtwald Hospice.
7. See also Müller and Kern (2002), who propose a model of integrating hospice and palliative services which is based on a situation very similar to the one described here.
8. By using this metaphor here and at few other occasions in the text, I just mean to say that something, like my field, is not a naturally delineated given. I do not intend to take a constructionist theoretical attitude in the stricter sense, with possibly far-reaching epistemological implications. For an overview of positions on this matter see Hacking (1999) and, with reference to medicine, Lupton (2000).
9. Reflexively reporting from a socially constitutive configuration aims at the 'situated knowledge' Donna Haraway (1988) proposes – a kind of knowledge that is neither universally objective in a traditional sense nor completely relativist.
10. Holmberg (2005), for example, presents interview material illustrating this point extremely well. Large-scale sociological surveys on awareness (e.g. Seale et al. 1997) tend to assume that 'awareness' is a constant mental state. From the point of view of long-term participant observation, this is not the case. For a differentiated discussion of the nurses' role in disclosing terminal illness, see May (1993).
11. Christine Pfeffer (1998: 14) seems to have adopted a very similar approach towards her role in fieldwork.
12. My postgraduate year in the U.K., where the NHS places great emphasis on research ethics procedures, may have been the most important influence here. For a U.K. perspective on research ethics in the hospice context see Lawton (2001).
13. Ultimately, I would agree with anthropologists like Gary Fine, who argue that ethical ambivalences are an essential, unavoidable and possibly desirable part of the practice of ethnography (Fine 1993).

3
AN ETHNOGRAPHIC ACCOUNT
OF EVERYDAY HOSPICE CARE

Hospital or Home? The Spatial and Figurative Setting
of Stadtwald Hospice

The outside perceptions about hospices with which I was confronted during my research were often quite inaccurate. The idea that a hospice was bound to be somehow morbid and very depressing seemed to be deeply rooted in my own social surrounding in a large city, consisting mainly of young adults with university education. During my work on this study, when someone asked me about the topic of my research, reactions to my reply were usually along the lines of 'That must be terribly depressing...', 'How can you deal with such experiences?' or 'Such research would really bring me down'.

On the other hand, there seemed to be a vague conviction that something was wrong with death in our society, and that there was some need for change: 'Interesting topic. Our society denies death, doesn't it?' was a very frequent type of reaction, and quite a number of people I talked to were quick to mention that a relative worked in the church parish's volunteer hospice, or that a friend studying psychology had done a university seminar about death, or the like.

When compared to nursing homes, hospitals and even doctors' practices I visited during my research, Stadtwald Hospice gave the impression of a friendly, positive and sometimes even lively place. Patients, relatives and visitors coming there for the first time often expressed their pleasant surprise. The occasion of my own first visit was a short guided tour of the hospice. In my ethnographic diaries, it reads as follows:

I come out of the elevator and find myself standing on a tastefully, colourfully but modestly furnished corridor [Ger.: Etage], very bright and open, a lot of glass, which hardly allows associations with a hospital ward. The people on this floor are wearing civilian clothing. A woman in her early forties approaches me to say hello, she is the secretary ... I am impressed by the pleasant atmosphere of the hospice, and say so.

My second visit was occasioned by a meeting with the manager of the hospice, in which we discussed my research project:

The colours are dark blue and ochre, many potted plants standing everywhere, on the floor as well, there is a scratching board [Ger.: Kratzbaum] and a sleeping basket for the cat. Death announcements are pinned on a board entitled 'Farewells', right next to it there is another bulletin board with announcements and course advertisements, for example a sign-up list for people who want to join an arts and crafts session in Advent. Below it a table, with leaflets spread out [Ger.: aufgefächert] on it. ... It all makes for a very tasteful, yet straightforward impression. Individual details – the robust carpet, a table that can be wiped clean – seem very functional and sober on closer inspection. In a small meeting room I sit at a table for about four people. Opposite me there is a bookshelf, where specialised medical literature, e.g. 'Pharmacological Therapy', stands beside works on consolation, folk wisdom and psychotherapy [Ger.: Trost-, Sprüche- und Therapieliteratur], such as 'Aromatherapeutic massage', the Bible, a book on how to handle corpses, I scribble down the titles. There are a few folders on the lowest level of the shelf, a plate with some coffee creamer and cups next to it. On the walls a few pictures: sunflowers, a Polish mountain signpost with arrows pointing in different directions, footprints in the sand. [...] A couple of slightly kitsch items [Ger.: ein paar Niedlichkeiten] are standing around on the bookshelves opposite: two cats on a park bench, a little clown doll.

The third time I visited, I was going to present my research proposal in the weekly assembly of all full-time nursing staff, called the team meeting, and I had to wait a while before I was asked to come into the meeting room:

Back in the staff room, she [an assistant nurse] tells me to wait a little, I ask whether it is OK to sit down, and have to remove a jumper from the chair in order to do so. She points out the mess apologetically: there are used champagne glasses on a tray on the table, with a note saying 'champagne in the fridge', there is a tea pot and some used coffee mugs, a patient file and some more stuff. I ask whether that is for a birthday or still for New Year; she says it is two patients' [Ger.: Patienten] birthdays. I am surprised that she does not say 'residents' [Ger.: Bewohner], as is customary in many German hospices, but it also somehow seems more honest to me. I sit down at the table. After a couple of minutes I notice that I am still holding on tightly to my file on my lap, and put it on the table. I say hello to a tall woman in a dressing gown who passes by, and some visitors who pass by say hello to me. ... Then I sit for a while and look at the room. In the front part, which is half separated by a glass pane, is a kind of miniature office, a small printer or photocopying machine stands on the desk. In the back part, where I am sitting, is some sort of a small kitchen. It seems difficult to tell about the precise function of the room. Again I find the colours and the furniture very pleasant and homey, things are brown, ochre, blue. ... On my left there is a small cart with patient files. I notice how my nursing internship has changed my perception: I know now that they are patient files, and I find myself comparing the relaxed, cosy but clean atmosphere in this room with that in the nursing home ward, which was very hygienic and totally impersonal. On the right is a large wardrobe, on it are manuals for the use of some sort of machinery that apparently tends to clog up: I guess anaesthetic pumps [Ger.: Schmerzpumpen] or the like. The wardrobe on my left is covered in little note stickers, which suggest it contains medicine and medical equipment, some dressing materials are lying on it nearer to the wall. On the chairs are items of clothing, a sweat-shirt, a woollen jacket. On one of the wardrobes hangs a poem, in which a fictional ninety-year-old admonishes the visitor always only to live for the day. 'Live for the day' [Ger. Lebe den Tag] is in bold print each time.

The descriptions show that pleasant aesthetic impressions were a dominant part of my own first experience of the hospice. In my diaries, it comes across as a spacious, comfortable place, its physical layout as colourful and varied, and I mention a variety of objects and impressions that I seem to have difficulty to put into clear nursing categories.

Described more systematically and from hindsight, the physical setting of the hospice was clearly functional. All rooms opened to one central corridor. On the one end of that corridor was the entrance area, which led to a large assembly room, staff toilets and visitor toilets, and then two offices, separated from the main corridor by large glass panes. From the entrance area, the main corridor could be accessed through a glass door. On one side the outside walls were again made of glass, and a wide view over the roofs of the city opened up. On that side, there were also several terraces. On the other side of the corridor, there were the patient rooms, always two single rooms sharing a bathroom. After a couple of patient rooms, there was the staff room and a meeting room, then more patient rooms, a large bath, the spacious communal kitchen and again patient rooms. While, on closer inspection, this physical pattern resembles a hospital ward layout quite accurately, the use of lots of glass and bright colours made that conclusion far from immediate for the visitor.

Additionally, the very functional general layout was decisively supplemented by aesthetically pleasing furnishing and decoration, which, on closer inspection, revealed two important figurative realms characterising Stadtwald Hospice: the first consisted of symbols and metaphors concerning life and was quite apparent to any perceptive observer. The second could more easily be discerned by visitors with some experience of the health system, such as patients, nurses, relatives or the researcher: it was a strong aesthetic and figurative emphasis on not being a hospital, a nursing home, or any other institution of the regular health system.[1]

When I first presented my own research project to staff in the team meeting mentioned above, a senior nurse predicted confidently that I would soon change my preliminary topic from 'Death in the Hospice' to 'Life in the Hospice'. So I did in due course. In the diary descriptions given above, an emphasis on life is evident, both in the form of representations of the human life course and in the form of biological life: plants and animals, and pictures, photographs and other representations of both could be found all over the ward. The hospice cat received much attention from many people present, and there was an artificial fountain in which a patient's sister had put several kinds of fish which she fed every day. One patient lived with her cat during her time at the hospice, and one of the doctors regularly brought his dog when he came to see patients. There were pictures of plants and animals on the placards displaying patients' names at their doors, and small puppets and other arts and crafts type representations of – mostly young and endearing – animals stood on bookshelves and in corners.

In fact, life in the form of animals and plants often occasioned patients' lived experience and created a multitude of small stories:

> Today, I am in Mrs Hansen's room when she gets a bouquet of flowers from one of her countless visitors. I go and get a slim porcelain vase from the vase cupboard; the bouquet consists of a rose with a little green. It is the eighth one that is now in her room. The visitor is enthusiastic about us having a cat, too, she likes that very much. Dr Jensen's dog is there as well. He gets cat food, but only once Dr Jensen has given him permission. I guess that is to make sure that he does not devour the cat's food each time.

In this small excerpt, the symbolic giving of flowers was taken to extremes by relatives of one patient, who achieved some prominence because of this, as her eight bouquets were mentioned in conversation for days. More importantly, however, the hospice cat typically occasioned a lot of affectionate feelings and was always worth a small conversation between patients, nurses and visitors.

Life metaphors of another kind were manifest in the pictures and texts hanging in the team room and in the meeting room: There, it was the trajectories of human life which were figuratively represented: a picture of a signpost in the mountains could be interpreted as orientation in difficult times of one's life, a photograph of footprints on the sand of a beach, with waves coming in, pointed to the frailty of human achievements during the course of life. The poem 'Live for the Day' showed an emphasis on the conscious experience of the small things in everyday life – a central topic I shall come back to at greater length later. Life was thus figuratively represented everywhere in the interiors of Stadtwald Hospice. At the time of my research, there were few walls in the public hospice areas without some item that could be interpreted as a life symbol or metaphor, be it a plant, a picture or some allusion to the course of human life.

The second area of figurative and aesthetic representation prominent in the accounts I have presented above concerned the distinction which the hospice claimed from hospitals and nursing homes: this began with the colour of the walls and floors, which were beige and blue respectively, while other institutions of the health system tend to be painted in white, grey or light green. The fact that the whole hospice had carpets on the floor, rather than the linoleum customary elsewhere, points to a different understanding of what is comfortable, but also to a lesser emphasis on hygiene: carpets may give a more homely atmosphere, but are relatively difficult to clean and need to be replaced more often than linoleum. An ostentatious difference in approaches to hygiene was also demonstrated by the presence of live animals and plants, which would be banned in many hospitals as possible carriers of germs.

All employees in the hospice wore plain clothes rather than nurses' uniforms, and the dominant hospital clothing colours, white and light green, were seen only rarely. Civilian clothes can be interpreted as an emphasis on individuality in the hospice, and suggest that institutional roles of different professional groups, and status differences within such groups, were either unimportant or consciously downplayed.

On the staff room bookshelves I previously described, different genres of writing were mixed, which suggests that there was no clear-cut hierarchy of biomedical, nursing, esoteric, psychotherapeutic and other knowledge, but rather – at least outwardly – an eclectic approach. In a similar fashion, objects from the professional area of nursing and administration (patient files), the private life of the patients (champagne glasses), and the nurses' work breaks (coffee cups) mixed freely on the table of the staff room, and the fact that this mixture was not immediately cleaned up and separated is only the last one in a chain of indications that points to an intermingling of categories which would ideally be kept separate in a classical hospital.

The emphasis on the difference from other institutions of the health system thus displayed at Stadtwald Hospice is all the more significant since such institutions provided the background from which almost all people in the hospice came: for the patients, hospitals had been the setting of much of their life during their illness trajectory, and for the nurses they were the place where their professional training and former professional life had taken place. The emphasis on distinction can thus neither be accidental, nor was it difficult to discern for the audience in question.

A meeting with a nurse seconded to the hospice for the first time by a temping agency shows this clearly:

Today there is a temping nurse, to improve staffing, she is called Marion and is wearing a blue overall as work clothes. She is a little dazzled by a number of things: on the one hand, I hand her the hospice brochure and she is astonished that an institution which has so little funding and relies on charity money is willing to afford a temping nurse. On the other hand, she is very surprised when the cat comes in and sniffs at her. She does not understand the fact that there are no distinct working clothes here either, and thinks at first that we work in our ordinary street clothes. When I explain that we use normal clothes as working clothes, but still distinguish clearly, she is puzzled, and says she has no old clothes which she does not wear otherwise.

The point here is not to claim that all hospitals are grey and all nursing homes unfriendly. Some may be, others are certainly not. Rather, it is important to realise that Stadtwald Hospice, in important aspects of its setting and practice, was designed in contradistinction from institutions that were perceived to be grey, impersonal and unfriendly. For daily life at the hospice, perceptions of hospitals and nursing homes were important, quite independent of their accuracy, which they sometimes had and sometimes did not have. This is clear in a conversation some nurses had about a local research hospital:

> Mrs Nitzke was admitted to Hoheneich Hospital Centre, diagnostic measures, nobody believes that there are still any chances to help her. There is vague talk about the possible point of it, until Ute says, well that's clear, they want to 'open her up', 'they do research there', 'it's a research hospital, you know'. Some more such expressions are used and nobody objects; it's just that Mrs Nitzke puts her hope in the hospital, as Sieglinde says with resignation. Apart from that, everybody seems to agree with Ute that Mrs Nitzke is being exploited for research, but it seems nobody wants to phrase it that drastically.

In this case, the patient returned after some days without any of the nurses' grim predictions having come true. In another, contrasting episode, a very well trained nurse gave me a detailed and credible account of how a patient had suffered some severe medical and mental setbacks from lack of attention in a hospital:

> Afterwards on the corridor I ask Walter what the point of a suprapubic catheter is; he says it is less infectious than one via the urethra. He explains some other things in Mr Kasparek's clinical picture [Ger.: Krankheitsbild] and, while he stays outwardly calm, he does get a bit worked up about it. He says he is angry because, in the hospital, quite a number of things had been done wrong with Mr Kasparek. First, the patient contracted a bladder infection, which could be detected by the particles in his urine, and something like that was completely superfluous. The way he phrases it, is sounds as if the hospital had actually made the bladder infection. Then, he was never mobilised, which gave him bedsores [on the lower back] and intestinal problems, because he had not been allowed to sit on the toilet, but been given strong laxatives and an incontinence pad instead. This in turn led to semi-liquid excrement [Ger.: schmieriger Stuhl], which of course was no good for the bedsores. Besides all this there were the psychological problems, which a situation like that caused for a man like him. It was now of crucial importance to mobilise him as often as possible, in order to make the bedsores go away and get to grips with the intestinal problem in a less aggressive fashion.

The hospice, of course, would try to set this right, and, in fact, the treatment regime of many patients was altered on arrival. Not without reason – hospice staff were, for example, extremely skilled in the treatment of bedsores and often cured bedsores that had plagued patients for a long time and had left doctors helpless in other institutions.

Perceptions of what hospitals or nursing homes were supposed to be like ranged from clothing and decoration to architectural layout. An interview partner from another German hospice once complained to me that the architectural layout of her hospice made it impossible to emphasise this distinction sufficiently. She mentioned that her hospice just could not compare with the Victorian mansions used elsewhere, clearly assuming that a 'real' hospice must not look like a hospital ward.

A bias against hospitals and nursing homes is of course highly likely to structure such perceptions; they were, on the one hand, mostly owed to nurses' personal experience in hospitals or nursing homes, and thus more than myth or bad publicity. However, those nurses who quite liked working in hospitals or nursing homes and who worked in exemplary ones probably never saw any reason to leave and work in a hospice. Perceptions, whatever the reality behind them, were an important element of institutional atmosphere at the hospice and, in that sense, very real.

There were telling symbolic distinctions in sets of rules – or their absence – and in standards of behaviour, too. In Stadtwald Hospice, patients were given an unusual amount of freedom in planning their day and choosing their activities. This was by no means just limited to a symbolic function, but still perceived as symbolic by the outside world since it was, again, in striking contrast to hospital rules. Patients were, for example, allowed to get up whenever they wanted to and to have their meals when they wanted to. They did not need to take all of their pills if they did not want to, even though they were usually very strongly encouraged to take their painkillers and their medication for digestion. They were allowed to smoke and to drink alcohol. While the hospice did not encourage drinking or smoking cannabis, and provided neither large amounts of alcohol nor any illicit drugs, it tolerated such practices as long as they did not interfere with the nurses' work or other patients' privacy.

In the communal kitchen, food was prepared individually in the same room where the patients and some staff ate, a practice violating several boundaries of standard hygiene procedures in medical institutions. Such practice was unheard of in standard healthcare contexts and viewed with great suspicion by supervising governmental medical authorities. During my fieldwork period, the hospice management had to engage in sympathetic, but very tough negotiations with these authorities concerning a number of issues in the field of hygiene, but also concerning hierarchy and accountability within the interdisciplinary nursing team.

When I first worked at Stadtwald Hospice, it also struck me that the nurses sometimes did not know what exact kind of cancer a patient had, even when patients had been in the hospice for some time. I realised soon that the biomedical diagnosis was only relevant for the nurses in so far it related to actual symptoms they were trying to alleviate. Where exactly the cancer had started, or what kind of cells it consisted of, often had no implications for hospice nursing at all. As a biomedical fact itself, it was not of much worth.

With reference to Mrs Röbeling, I try a number of times to ask what exactly it is one dies from in the case of leukaemia. The nurses never quite tell me, they somehow seem to find the question makes no sense, or is irrelevant. Maria has not even understood what I mean: she says cancer of the blood, leukaemia is cancer of the blood. I know that. Today I ask Lena, who does not quite know either, and mentions it at handover. Infections maybe, somebody says, they do not know what to say, the white blood cells eat the red ones, somebody else suggests; I get a little embarrassed and content myself with that. Renate [a senior nurse] surely knows, I am assured. Maybe it is because dying in the end is so similar that it becomes irrelevant what one is exactly dying from. This view would be supported by the fact that the nurses often do not know what kind of cancer it is that somebody has, and that this does not seem to be too important for them, either. I suppose what one dies from is 'multiple organ failure' and general weakness. The only concrete thing I have heard so far is suffocation, and that of course has very negative connotations. Once it was mentioned that cancer of the brain can put pressure on the breathing centre and thus lead to death.

Since the aims of hospice care were palliative rather than curative, its focus was the lived experience of the patient rather than the biomedical therapy of the body. The criterion for treatment was whether it would improve patients' experience, and the biomedical diagnosis was often not important for this anymore. In this physical respect, the 'medical gaze' (Foucault 1991[1963]) on the patient's body had been suspended – I shall come back to its continuing relevance concerning the patient's personality and emotions at a later point.

In conclusion, two points are of more general relevance: first, there is a close connection between emphasising life and distinguishing hospice practice from that of hospitals and nursing homes. The underlying general assumption was that most other, standard healthcare institutions made it impossible for their patients to experience their life, or at least significant parts of it, as meaningful. The hospice, in its symbolic presentation, emphasised life because this was seen as distinct from the hospital (or nursing home) experience and, vice versa, it distanced itself from hospitals and nursing homes because those were perceived as places that were not conducive to meaningful life experience. In this way, the figurative emphasis on life and the distinction from other institutions of the health system are certainly closely connected.

On a higher level of figurative organisation, most of the images, metaphors and symbolic practices discussed so far can be related to an overarching summary image, namely that of the private household. The household image, containing associations such as individuality, familiarity, privacy, flexibility, emotional warmth, sociality and ultimately life, and making them available through the symbols, metaphors and practices described above, was implemented in Stadtwald Hospice in contradistinction to the image of the public healthcare institution, related to categories and feelings such as conformity, anonymity, loneliness, structure, scientific rationality and social (and ultimately biological) death. Of course, such implementation was not uniform and always precarious in the face of administrative and organisational pressures, as will be shown later.[2]

James Fernandez (1986) has emphasised that people are persuaded through metaphorical predication and figurative thinking to take on identities, and that identities thus acquired may engender social performances. The function of household imagery in Stadtwald Hospice can be analysed in these two directions: On the one hand, it continuously invited patients, nurses and visitors to be persuaded to take on a positive identity in relation to the hospice. The identification 'I am a household member' implies a range of sentiments like feeling looked after, at ease, connected, at home, or the like. On the other hand, the image also provided a goal to implement in performance, to fulfil the household member's role, to be responsible, take initiatives, be content with emotional rewards, etc. Role expectations like 'I shall work/live/visit here as I would in a home, not in an institution', or similar ones, offer themselves and point towards active performances of a certain kind. The image of the private household is an organising category that can serve as an excellent background for a more detailed discussion of hospice life in the following chapters.[3]

Good Hospice Care – A Discussion of Daily Nursing Practice

The distinction from hospitals and nursing homes, an emphasis on life as lived, and efforts to put the household image into practice extended far into the daily routines of hospice care. The aim of the next part of this study is to give a detailed account of that form of care. At the same time, it will pursue the closely related questions as to what the hospice understanding of good nursing care was about, which values became apparent in such practice and how hospice care was perceived to be different from practices in other institutions. At some points, the analysis draws inspiration from Goffman's (1959, 1985[1963]) work on stigma and on social roles in regard to their settings, but does not follow his approach rigidly.

My colleagues in 'the Care' ('die Pflege'), as German nurses call their professional world, were nurses of different specialisations with different degrees of qualification, ranging from a six-week Red Cross course like my own, to full-time, three-year training plus twenty years of experience and additional specialist training in oncology.[4] At any time, there were also student nurses, civilian service workers and some volunteers around.

Three shifts structured the day of nurses and patients. Morning shift, in which there was the most work to do, took place from 7 a.m. to 3.15 p.m., evening shift from 2.15 p.m. until 10.30 p.m., and night shift from 10 p.m. to 7.30 a.m. Morning shift was mostly staffed by five or six people, evening shift by four or five, night shift by two. With fifteen places for patients, the nurse: patient ratio was thus very generous by the standards of other institutions. Each shift began and ended with a handover – a meeting in which the most important events of the previous shift were discussed in detail with the incoming staff by those just finishing their shift.

Each shift had a marked rhythm, depending on the daily routines of the patients. This rhythm was never quite the same, since patients were allowed to get up and have breakfast whenever they wanted to, and all subsequent routines of the day varied accordingly. The resulting rhythm of the shift was the main organisational feature of the nurses' experience of their work, determining whether they could be relaxed or not at a given time, and whether it was a hectic, a quiet or maybe an 'unusual' shift.

On every shift, 'the examined' (Ger.: 'die Examinierten'), that is, fully trained nurses, were responsible for a number of patients. The other staff supported these senior nurses and had simpler nursing tasks delegated to them. My own area of work was what was referred to as basic care (Ger.: 'Grundpflege'), as distinguished from therapeutic care (Ger.: 'Behandlungspflege'). Basic care included helping patients with meals and with personal hygiene, including the management of incontinence, assisting nurses in more specialised tasks and running all sorts of errands.

The work life of the nurses was organised around the staff room, situated in the middle of the long central corridor. Medicine, patients' files and other important documentation were all kept here, the handover took place there, and so did shorter coffee breaks. In the staff room, nurses exchanged information concerning patients, planned their interaction with patients, relaxed in between seeing patients and had most of their meals. There they received call signals when patients wanted or needed something and there they answered incoming phone calls. At the same time, they could be informal and off guard in the staff room, plan all interactions with patients and assemble the material they would need. In spatial terms, going back and forth between the staff room and patients' rooms was what nursing was all about. In Goffman's (1959) terms, the staff room was the place where the nurses were 'backstage' in relation to patients, visitors and relatives, and none of those people were allowed to enter that room. Doctors, the manager and administrative staff could, however, enter whenever they wanted and sometimes stayed for a while on their own business.

What daily nursing routines were like in detail is probably best explained by illustrating the above remarks with examples from my interaction with five patients: Mr Rathje, Mrs Öttinger, Mrs Brunnhofer, Hans Dornschuh who has been mentioned before, and Mrs Behrens, as written down in my diaries. All five had different forms of cancer and were at different points in their illness trajectory when I met them, and yet, in different ways, the varying treatment of all of them represents a lot of what hospice care was about.

'I Have Been Looking For You...' – Helping Mr Rathje to Get Up

The starting point of hospice care was patients' bodies, and nurses engaging with them in a variety of ways. Deborah Lupton (2000: 57) aptly summarises the significance of the body in contemporary Western societies and its relation to notions of self: 'For the late modern individual, the body is seen as signifying the self, and demonstrating one's capacity for self-knowledge, self-mastery, and self-care. The ideal body is that which is tightly contained, its boundaries stringently policed, its orifices shut, kept autonomous, private and separate from other things and other bodies'. Each single aspect of the above paradigm is put in question by advanced cancer.

Julia Lawton, in her study of an English hospice, has even argued that 'inpatient hospices act as liminal spaces in which the unbounded body is both mediated and contained' (2000: 134), and provided ample evidence for the close connection between selfhood and containment of bodily fluids in the hospice context (1998, 2000: 122–47). Certainly, such containment was a central nursing practice at Stadtwald Hospice, too. In my own discussion of daily nursing practice, however, I would like to emphasise that nurses' dealings with patients were never only about bodies and their containment, but always located in a very complex web of emotion and communication about all sorts of things, and in the very practical work setting of nurses' routines. It is, I think, very important to discuss self and personhood in the context of the minute daily practices which constitute them, and while there were certainly a few extremely discomforting cases of total and humiliating bodily breakdown during the time of my fieldwork, it would not do justice to life at Stadtwald Hospice to present these in isolation.

My account of Mr Rathje, a patient I knew for quite some time while working at the hospice, starts with a description of him, which is quite representative of the hospice ways, in that an almost identical description of him in a very similar style could easily have been given at handover, introducing him to a nurse who had not met him before.

Mr Rathje is around sixty and suffers from a brain tumour. He is a small, but heavily built man and has the typical short, thin hair after head surgery and radiotherapy. His vision seems impaired; we are not sure how much he can still see. He cannot sit up in bed on his own and he is only able to stand up and remain standing with assistance. He answers questions with yes or no, sometimes with short sentences. One can never tell for sure what exactly he still notices in his surroundings. He never says anything on his own initiative. Sometimes he smiles. At meals, one has to put the feeding cup into his hand, or a fork with food, and then he puts it into his mouth by himself. When he does not want any more, he passes the cup or the fork to the left into the void. ... Often, he just wants to sit somewhere, in the kitchen or on the corridor, not in his room. When he is there, the door is mostly open.

At handover, such a description would, in addition, typically have included the exact medication and details of treatment and, if applicable, have mentioned whether medical apparatus such as a special mattress was used. It would have mentioned what the patient knew about his illness ('Mr Rathje has been informed about his condition...') some personal preferences of food or leisure ('Mr Rathje likes red wine and watches the evening news...') and finally his psychological situation ('Mr Rathje is quite resigned...', or: 'Mr Rathje is very troubled by the fact that he needs help...').

Mr Rathje needed help in all aspects of daily life. In the hospice, such tasks were combined into regular routines, such as the morning routine, and nurses who knew the relevant routines of a patient were, in their own jargon, said to know 'the care of somebody' (Ger.: die Pflege von jemand kennen). In the case of Mr Rathje, I knew the relevant routines and had, on the day in question, been delegated the task of looking after him while the senior nurse in charge worked next door and helped me occasionally.

> A little after handover Hannah approaches me and says Mr Rathje is awake. Yesterday, he had slept until 1 p.m., and therefore the nightshift did not give him any sleeping pills this time. Hannah tells me to wash him, how thoroughly, I ask, all over, or just refresh him a little? Then an idea comes to my mind, maybe a shower? Hannah also hesitates a little and then says, maybe we should let him have a shower, that is what I just thought, I say. We have a look in his file: his last shower was five days ago, so one is due today. I go to his room and say, good morning, what about a shower before breakfast, Mr Rathje, that would be OK, wouldn't it? Yes, he says firmly, I have already been looking for you. I smile inwardly about this way of confirmation: Mr Rathje is not able to go looking for me, and talks little at other times, so I am content that the prospect of having a shower seems to have such a positive effect on him, making him talk at such length.

Mr Rathje could determine by himself the time when he would get up – a nurse would just check occasionally whether he was awake. However, that freedom was already severely limited by medication and his limited control over his body. In actual fact, once he was awake, he depended totally on somebody who would help him to get up. In principle, Mr Rathje was asked to decide by himself how to go about his personal hygiene, but the suggestive question I put to him in the diary excerpt concerning showers is quite typical: it was motivated by the necessity to coordinate one patient's needs with those of others, and of course by the hygienic rule that regular showers are advisable. So while there was a general willingness to let Mr Rathje decide how he wanted to go about the beginning of this day, to carry out even the most basic tasks resulting from his decisions was already mostly outside his influence.

Originally, the plan to let Mr Rathje have a shower was decided upon when the nurses looked for the relevant information in his patient file and found it. Interaction with Mr Rathje – as with any patient – was accompanied by a dense and continuous flow of information. This was passed on orally at handover on the one hand, and in the documentation of Mr Rathje's illness in his file on the other. We, the nurses, knew when he had had his last shower, how his mood had been three days ago, whether he had taken his pills the day before or when he last defecated. If we did not know, we were in a position to find out quickly. Mr Rathje himself may, in fact, easily not have remembered any of this; the decisive information lay with the nurses. The founders of the hospice had envisaged handover to take place by the patients' bedside, but I was told that this practice had proven to be too time-consuming and impractical.

So I get a shower chair [Ger.: Duschstuhl; a robust chair with small wheels and a hole in the middle of the seat] from the ward bathroom, and some new towels. Then I pop into Mr Rathje's bathroom, let the shower run until it is warm, and put the heating on. Then I stand on the left of his bed, and Hannah on the right; we let the bed move upwards a little bit [beds can be moved electrically], take the duvet away, and ask Mr Rathje to let go of the bell cord [for calling the nurse] to which he is holding on tightly over his chest. First, we take off his T-Shirt – he can still help with the arms – then we straighten him up in bed into a sitting position, with his help, until he sits on the edge of the bed. He needs to be supported in all this. Now he gets his shoes put on. In between, we tell him as usual about what we are going to do next, or praise him for his help and thank him for it. Then I lift him into a standing position and Hannah takes the incontinence pad away; some dark liquid excrement is on it. I am surprised not to find any urine in it, yesterday there was a lot and he has drunk well [Ger.: er hatte gut getrunken]. Then Mr Rathje, very slowly and a little unsteadily, takes three steps in a circle and, always with my help, sits down on the shower chair.

Hospice care as I witnessed and practised it was characterised by addressing the patient continuously – in many cases almost independent of his capacity to reply, or to understand. My diaries just summarise this fact every now and then, but every little step of nursing procedure was likely to be accompanied by the nurse asking permission to do something, explaining something or asking the patient to do something.

In the present case, there is a degree of ambivalence. We could not really know what Mr Rathje understood at all. Even assuming that he did, we could not be sure whether he was at all capable of clear reasoning, and of replying. All this shows two aspects of ideas of the person underlying hospice practice: on the one hand, patients should be informed and put in a position to make their own decisions about everyday matters. The underlying ideal was that of a conscious, informed actor making choices. On the other hand, the conversational construction of a fully conscious person can also be interpreted as a strategy the nurses used to shield themselves from the fact that some of the patients they were dealing with – not Mr Rathje – may have been in an irrevocably unconscious state, sometimes almost brain-dead, to use drastic biomedical terms.

Another routine very typical of nursing in a hospice situation, which is recounted in the diary excerpt, was the matter of fact handling and control of faeces and urine by the nurses. Almost all patients became incontinent at least during the last days of their fatal illness, and for many this started weeks before their eventual death. Apart from general weakness and loss of control over the body, the functioning of the digestive system is slowed down by the side effects of painkillers. As a consequence, it needed to be monitored closely to prevent a closure of the digestive tract, which has extremely unpleasant consequences for patients. So the use and handling of different forms of incontinence pads, and the monitoring of what was found, was a standard nursing routine, maybe the one that was performed most often.

Both practices, addressing the patient all the time, and handling and monitoring faeces and urine in a casual, passing fashion, continue throughout the account I give of Mr Rathje having a shower and getting dressed in the morning.

Hannah says we still need to get a faeces pot [Ger.: Fäkalientopf] to insert into the shower chair. I do that, while she pushes the chair with Mr Rathje into the shower. I put the pot underneath him and put the shower on. Showering his hand a little, I ask him whether that is the right temperature. Yes, he says. I put the shower head into his hand and tell him to go on and shower himself everywhere he is able to reach. He can do it quite well today and seems to like having a shower.

Meanwhile, I have noticed that there are still faeces on his scrotum and his behind, so I go and get a plastic glove for myself. Mr Rathje showers on his own, apart from the back of the head and the back, where I help him. I also assist with the soap, because he seems to be unable to relate to the shower gel I put in his palm. Then I hand him a towel for his head, so he can start to dry himself in order not to get cold, and I get myself a flannel for [cleaning] his behind and genitals. The first flannel ends up covered in faeces, the second one still a little. While washing him, I feel more, firmer excrements coming, and let that happen – it happens frequently when patients get from a lying into a sitting position. With a splash, it falls into the pot, which has half filled with water, twice. Later I tell Hannah, Mr Rathje has defecated once more, oh how nice, she says, quite pleased.

In the meantime, Hannah has made the bed in the room and brought a wheelchair. Then we get to the transfer from the shower stool into the wheelchair. We position the wheelchair just outside the bathroom door, when I notice that Mr Rathje is urinating onto the floor and the wheels of the shower stool. We just take notice of it, and I am aware at that moment how very unusual it would be for outsiders to observe our calmness. When he has finished, Hannah puts a towel between the backrest of the shower stool, which is wet from the shower water, and the back of Mr Rathje, which should now remain dry. I ask Mr Rathje again whether he is cold, yes, he says, now I am. I ask Hannah to get a fresh T-Shirt quickly, and while they put it on I wipe his bottom once more with a large handful of toilet paper.

We put his socks on him and start to put his trousers over his feet, so we can just lift them up later. Then we wheel him to the wash basin, to which he holds on and lifts himself up, with us supporting him on both arms. While he is standing, Hannah wipes his bottom with an oil against bedsores, we put a new incontinence pad on him and pull up the trousers we prepared before. Then we exchange the shower stool for a wheelchair and he sits down again. I wheel him into his room, quickly flood the shower floor with water, put the faeces pot into the room, where Hannah takes it away, and shave Mr Rathje with his electric shaver. Then I wheel him to the kitchen for breakfast. (...) I have quite a harmonious feeling about the procedure with Mr Rathje: he was able to do a lot of things on his own, he was in a good mood, there were no complications and the atmosphere was relaxed.

The morning routine of Mr Rathje, an essential part of 'his care', ends here. Several tasks of hospice nursing were completed: we helped the patient to change his incontinence pads, to get up, to have a shower and to get dressed. He was sat in a wheelchair and thus, in nursing jargon, 'mobilised'. Shaving, washing, getting dressed, incontinence pad and wheelchair make it possible for Mr Rathje to participate in the social interaction possibly awaiting him at breakfast in the communal kitchen.

Mary Douglas has pointed out how 'We should expect the orifices of the body to symbolise its specially vulnerable points. Matter issuing from them is marginal stuff of the most obvious kind' (Douglas 2002[1966]: 150). This view makes it possible to explain the nature of the stigma in question, and its management, in greater depth. The nurses' work, then, is to eradicate all signs of such marginal stuff having passed through the boundaries of the body. Two stigmatising effects can thus be concealed: first, the very fact of the appearance of marginal matter – faeces, urine, beard stubble and sweat are considered indecent. Second, nurses' work also aims at pretending to the world outside of the bathroom that the patient has more control of his body than he really has, loss of control of the body itself being seen as a stigma in contemporary society: 'Ill, disabled or dying people are the "other", those from whom the healthy, young and able-bodied seek, often unconsciously, to differentiate themselves because of the fears, anxieties, revulsion and dread they harbour of the incipient chaos and dissolution of their own bodies' (Lupton 2000: 58). It is the nurses' work to create at least a partial illusion of specific and general bodily normality when preparing a patient for social interaction.[5]

This projection of social interaction at breakfast is also worth pointing out because Mr Rathje in fact never communicated with any other patients while I knew him and he possibly did not even notice them. At the most, he exchanged an occasional remark with the person helping him to eat, or with his wife, who came to visit every day. In principle, he could have stayed in bed and have had breakfast there, and in other institutions with less personnel this would have been the normal procedure to follow. However, in the hospice framework, it was quite typical that a patient's possibility to interact with others and to have new experiences was judged more important than the time efficiency of nursing routines. He was prepared for such a social role as long as there was any possibility that he might want it, or want to re-establish it.

While we attempted at all times to communicate with Mr Rathje, it was often unclear what he really would have wanted, and without our assistance he would have remained helpless and most probably hardly have expressed any wishes. All routines were ultimately dominated by us nurses. The question as to whether he welcomed the individual steps of his treatment by us has to remain largely unanswered, the only statement he made initially was that he would like a shower. Since a routine like the one described happened every day, it could be interpreted as normal that the patient did not comment on it. In any case, ample occasion for communication was given and we assumed at all times that he was conscious, informed, and somewhat eager for social interaction and non-standard experiences – a normal adult personality of our own cultural background, just hindered in exercising his personal preferences by his progressing illness.

Concluding the presentation of Mr Rathje's case, I would like to pay some attention to another very important area of nursing routine, namely assisting patients with eating. I describe in my diaries how, on the same day, I helped Mr Rathje to have coffee and cake, which was routinely distributed at 3.30 p.m. every day.

> When I go to Mr Rathje he is sitting in his chair at the table in his room, leaning to one side as always. I ask him whether he wants coffee and cake; there is no reaction. I split the question: Do you want coffee? Yes. With milk? Yes. Sugar? Yes. A piece of cake? Yes. I get everything from the trolley and tell Rüdiger [the civilian service worker with whom I am working] that I am going to help Mr Rathje. Then I sit down beside him, cut the cake into small pieces, open the feeding cup so the coffee can get a little colder, and put a piece of cake on the fork. I put it in his hand. He keeps it on his lap – no other reaction. Mr Rathje, there is a piece of cake on the fork. No reaction. Otherwise I can just give it to you. I take the fork away from him and put the cake to his mouth, he eats and chews slowly. His eyes are a little bloodshot and even less open than usual. Are you tired, Mr Rathje? Yes, he says. I give him another little piece of cake, which he again chews very slowly, then I put the feeding cup into his hand once again, he drinks a little sip. Then he does not react at all any more and seems totally absent, the fork resting in his hand on his lap. Have you had enough, I ask. Yes, says Mr Rathje. I start putting things away. Do you want to sit on the chair or go to bed? Rather in the chair? Yes. I walk out of the room and look at my watch in passing. I was in his room for twenty minutes.

In the excerpt, communication with Mr Rathje was hardly possible. While looking after him, I had the impression that questions asking for a decision of the type 'A or B' were too much for him, and I started to ask questions that could be answered with 'Yes' or 'No'. At first, I tried to motivate him to eat, until I felt safe to conclude that he was really not very interested.

Again, this shows that hospice nursing tried to assume as much patient interest in everyday activities as possible. Intact mental capabilities of the patient were also assumed as a matter of fact, sometimes regardless of whether there had been actual evidence of them: the whole situation described assumes that Mr Rathje has an accurate judgement of the situation and his own desires. Finally, the time frame used is significant: for most hospitals or nursing homes, it would be rather unusual for a member of staff to spend such a long time trying to find out whether or not a patient with all sorts of severe restrictions wanted to eat his cake.

Additionally, it is helpful here to pick up the earlier discussion of matter passing in and out of patients' bodies, this time in relation to eating and drinking. McInerney (1992) has discussed the provision of food and fluids in terminal care and points out how food and fluids are strongly associated with life in such contexts, even once they have become irrelevant from the biomedical point of view. Seen this way, what I was engaging in as a nurse when insisting on giving a patient food and drink was a symbolic interaction denoting life, in line with hospice symbolism discussed earlier. This may be quite independent from the question of whether or not the patient actually wants or needs to eat or drink.

Mr Rathje was, in many respects, quite a typical hospice patient, and so my interactions with him are to some degree quite representative for interaction with other patients. As he was limited in movement, control over his bodily functions, expression and possibly cognition, so were very many cancer patients in the last weeks of their terminal illness. The underlying assumption of my interaction with him was, however, that until definite proof to the contrary, it had to be assumed that he basically had cognition, intentions and desires hardly different from those of healthy adults, just buried underneath the outward signs of his illness.

'One Cannot Think about the Illness All the Time' – Breakfast For Mrs Öttinger

Mrs Öttinger was an elderly woman of eighty-eight years, suffering from stomach cancer, who came to the hospice after a fall in her own apartment that had left her confused and hardly able to move. By the time I got to know her, however, Mrs Öttinger had made a remarkable recovery not untypical of elderly patients who are looked after with care and attention. Even though she was quite weak, she walked shorter distances by herself, organised her daily activities by herself, was fully conscious and aware of her surroundings, and clearly aware of her terminal diagnosis. The only help she needed was some assistance with her morning routines and showers, and some company. My dealings with her display a set of hospice nursing approaches which are, on the surface, different from those described above. I will attempt to show, however, that underlying attitudes are quite similar.

45

Today, I am responsible for Mrs Öttinger again, as in the last couple of days. This starts by going into her room at 7.50 a.m. and putting her medicine there; she is still asleep, I take some dirty dishes with me. At 8.20 a.m. I look in again: she is dozing. I wish her a good morning and point the medicine out to her, which is a formality really: I know she will first go to breakfast by herself, then rest a while, and only then start her morning routine, for which she needs my help. But I want to make contact with her and know how she is feeling today and what her plans are. I take the lid off the drops, which she cannot do by herself, and she tells me that she ate almost a whole jar of pickled pumpkin during the night, which she shows me. She says she is sorry now that yesterday evening's fruit is still standing around. I suggest to tell the kitchen that she likes sour things; she says the kitchen knows that already, and she always has some guerkins with dinner. We make an appointment, as is customary with mostly independent patients: she says she will first have breakfast and then rest a little, yes, and then we could do the morning routine. If you want, I say, well, she says, it could be that the physiotherapist comes, then she would rest afterwards, it will depend on that. OK, I say, I will come again in three-quarters of an hour and have a look who is first, me or the physio. But then it's your own breakfast time, she points out, we will see, I reply. Then I go and get a clean glass from the kitchen, because she is very thirsty, and bring the paper with me. The sticker 'Morning News please' from her door has gone and I offer to make a new one, but then I discover the sticker on the wardrobe and stick it on the door again. Then I say goodbye. When I come back three-quarters of an hour later the physio is there; I exchange a few words with both of them and say, I will be back in an hour.

The previously discussed patient, Mr Rathje, was put in a position where, theoretically, he would have been able to take charge of his affairs. He was, however, unable to do so. A similar approach was taken in my dealings with Mrs Öttinger, and, in contrast with Mr Rathje, she had quite clear ideas and was well able to follow up a number of them by herself: she got up when she wanted to, had breakfast when she wanted to, and synchronised all this with her appointment with the physiotherapist and her desire for a nap afterwards. The morning routine and my help with it was the most flexible item in her morning plans, but she in turn took the staff breakfast times into consideration. In the end, I had to make several attempts to synchronise my own schedule with hers and to negotiate the times of our morning routine together, always trying to find out what would suit her best. I contacted her three times until we finally came to a definite agreement. Meanwhile, we chatted a little and I fixed some things in her room. On re-reading my diary, it struck me that my role seemed almost like that of a personal servant, rather than that of an assistant nurse.

The morning routine also took on a form quite different from that of Mr Rathje. My role was just to be present in case help was needed and to assist her with the few things she could not do by herself, but she was fully in charge of what was being done, at what time and in which order:

After our breakfast, I go to Mrs Öttinger again. She is sitting on the edge of the bed, and almost seems to be waiting for me. She goes to the bathroom by herself and does not really need so much help. I make her bed while she washes, hand her some stuff in between, dry her back and get a fresh towel. While drying her back I massage the muscles a little, which is good for her, she says. She has an exact routine of which clothes to put where, whether to air them or to put them on the chair overnight, and in which order she puts them on. She wears a truss, because her belly bulges out enormously – a mixture of hernia, ruptured old scars and her stomach cancer.

Mrs Öttinger was also quite aware of her illness situation and, in her daily life, consciously tried to develop little routines and coping strategies to deal with it:

She tells me how she sends her nephew, who lives in a supervised living project [Ger.: betreute Wohngruppe], rhymed postcards, he has nobody else. Postcards with horses on them are especially good; one she got from Sieglinde; she shows it to me. In fact, a horse is put out to grass on the grounds of the supervised living project. She tells me of four old schoolmates of hers, with whom she is now exchanging letters again in old age, and she reads the rhymed text on the postcard to me. I ask whether she has been making these rhymes for a long time. No, she says, she had that idea here, because of the boredom. One has to be happy about small things and must not think about the illness all day, she adds. She is happy about the little things that the women from the arts and crafts group have brought her. They have given her two little snow men, an Easter egg, and a tile with egg and feather motifs on it.

In some ways, Mrs Öttinger clearly benefited from the opportunities for interaction, activity and the appreciation of daily life that the hospice offered. She enjoyed the possibility to chose from different types of food and she liked the small toy-like puppets made by the arts and crafts volunteer group of the hospice. She also got to know several other patients with whom she became friends as much as their respective limitations allowed. This is illustrated in one little story with romantic overtones, which she mentioned to me several times:

She also shows me a small doll, it is from somebody who passed away, his daughter has given it to her. They were friends, she tells me, he was ninety-four already, and always told his daughter, his little friend would come to visit him, and so the daughter gave her this as a memory [when he had died]. Of course, Mr Kühn, I say, yes, did you know him, she asks. He could not hear, so she tells me how they communicated through little notes, and they always sat together at mealtimes, she points out. I remember now that it had been mentioned that Mrs Öttinger was present at the Farewell [the farewell ritual often organised by hospice staff when a patient had died, see chapter six] for Mr Kühn.

Mrs Öttinger mentioned to me several times that it took a lot of discipline for her to go on, and she sometimes pondered why some people took longer to die than others. It would probably be mistaken to portray her as happy. The hospice, by providing people, attention, and the simple things and changes she needed for her coping, helped her to structure her days in a way that did not leave her totally exposed to the loneliness and boredom at home. She responded to this by being a demanding, but extremely thankful patient, who continuously stressed how much she liked life in the hospice.

One more thing about Mrs Öttinger made her case remarkable. During her stay in the hospice, she became – at least for her own standards – a small media celebrity. There was a euthanasia debate raging in the media at the time, and being almost the only patient in the hospice who was both willing and able to talk to the press and to TV teams, there was an article about her in the local press, and an interview was broadcast by a local radio station. Mrs Öttinger saw her role in this as that of a performer, and her goal was to convince journalists and their and audiences that the hospice was a great institution worthy of all support that could possibly be given. She said she had been trained to perform before, by her doctor, when they wanted to convince medical authorities to raise her nursing allowance, presenting her as frailer than she was. She mentioned to me that she tried hard not to say a single negative thing about the hospice when talking to journalists, and she also told me before an interview I myself did with her that she would of course only say good things, and the few critical points about the hospice were hardly worth mention in her opinion, and I should not mention them either.

This of course throws some light on the representation of hospice life to the outside public – and to scientific audiences. Both the media and researchers have mostly been interested in interviewing patients who were, like Mrs Öttinger, willing and able to talk about their situation. They have been much less interested in looking at daily nursing routines. In my experience, however, there were, at any given time, at the most two or three patients out of fifteen with whom interviews could possibly have been conducted. All others were too ill, unaware of their terminal condition, not outspoken enough or simply not interested in talking. A strong emphasis on interviewing as the main research method has certainly created a distortion in representations of hospice life, with patients being shown as far more conscious, aware and accessible than most are in everyday routines.[6]

Such an emphasis has also contributed to an idea – and may have been motivated by it in the first place – that impending death prompts people to think about their situation in a systematic way, to contemplate their lives, philosophy and religion. I had held this idea myself initially, but in my fieldwork experience, most hospice patients were almost exclusively interested in continuing their life patterns and maybe telling some life stories. Some discussed problems that had arisen over the years in relation to their family and those they felt close to. Hardly anybody was interested in religion, psychology, philosophy or other abstract sense-making systems. In cases where reflection on abstract matters had been part of earlier life patterns, it was maybe continued in the hospice, but where it had not been, it was hardly ever taken up.

There is, of course, a marked contrast in my accounts of Mr Rathje and Mrs Öttinger. One patient was mobile, aware, clearly conscious and could almost look after herself; for the other, the contrary was the case. The amount of help they needed, the treatment they received from nurses, and the amount and character of the interaction with staff differed accordingly. However, I argue that my approach as nurse had some common characteristics in both cases. Everyday tasks, such as helping patients to get up, to wash or to eat, were characterised most of all by an activating attitude that tried to put the patient in charge of her affairs and left as many aspects of daily life as possible to the patient to decide – even when she was hardly able to. In such cases, hospice nursing tried to fill in the gaps progressing cancer caused in the abilities of patients.

Both cases presented above represent extremes of that approach. In the case of Mr Rathje, the continuous offer to do things he was hardly able to do alone and to decide things of which he was perhaps not clearly conscious may seem slightly exaggerated to the outsider. In the case of Mrs Öttinger, my extreme flexibility in going along with her time planning will definitely seem luxurious and strange to a seasoned hospital nurse regularly working in understaffed shifts. In both cases, however, nurses' everyday actions were designed to facilitate a life that was as autonomous and self-reliant as the patient's situation allowed. Nursing was to be supplementary, help only given when a patient could not help herself.

Fading Life – Mrs Brunnhofer's Last Year

In the overall six months of my fieldwork, I got to know about one hundred hospice patients, and all except four of them died in the hospice. Those four, after some time at the hospice, got well enough to go home again, but died there shortly afterwards. Not surprisingly, death was the point to which all patients' stories converged. However, individual illness trajectories and patients' perspectives on their own situation were very different from each other. Some patients died only hours after they had been admitted; others stayed for almost a year. Some were clearly afflicted by a killing disease; others could have walked down the street without outward signs of illness – and in fact did do so. Some were fully aware that they were going to die soon; others planned the summer holiday almost until the end. What they all had in common, though, what characterised their illness experience and structured the care they needed, was the progression of their illness towards death and the changes that accompanied such a progression.

The disciplinary perspective of medicine, much criticised in this respect, would primarily describe this process as physical decline and progressing illness. Sociologists, from their discipline's vantage point, have called it 'fall from culture' (Seale 1998:149f). I find both approaches problematic in that they strongly prioritise the theoretical orientation of their discipline over the experience of nurses and patients. The ambiguous term 'deteriorating health' is problematic in this context, too. For most hospice patients, 'health' was a term from years past, and for the hospice staff, as has been pointed out, the emphasis of their work was on facilitating positive experience and ultimately life, not health.

From an ethnographic point of view, there is no ideal term to describe the process of change that goes on in the last weeks of dying from cancer. In order to avoid disciplinary prefigurations, I will use the broad expression 'fading of life', because that characterises patients' situations, nurses' experience with patients and my own ethnographic perspective as accurately as possible. I will use 'life' in the expression 'fading life' as a summary term for such analytical sub-categories as 'body', 'culture', 'health', 'mind' and 'personality', all bound to end with death, and I will use 'fading' to mean a loss of energy, vigour and interest in all these realms, and of their overall coherence. Different aspects of all of these were affected in different ways in individual patients, and, while there may be vagueness in my usage, it makes some degree of generalisation possible, and suits the ethnographic perspective of my work.

So, what faded when life faded? The physical strength of patients of course diminished all the time, and that was the most striking outward sign of impending death. However, together with that, sensory perception often decreased in power, patients went blind, could not taste or smell, lost appetite, had their perception covered over by painkillers, or their nerves blocked by cancer. Cancers or secondary growths in the brain could also lead to what I perceived as a fragmentation of some patients' personality: they lost parts or all of their memory, their character and moods changed significantly, their control of language and powers of expression were severely restricted, cognition as such became faulty and people were confused. Their general interest in the world, in pursuing activities and doing things, also often faded – not necessarily in immediate direct proportion to physical change – sometimes ahead of it, sometimes later.

In practical terms, it was often unclear what individual patients could still perceive, whether or not they had gone blind, if they could still talk and hear, and whether their immobility was due to paralysis or a lack of motivation to get up. It was sometimes hardly possible to tell whether a patient was addressing a nurse or talking to himself, and whether his bad mood was due to medication, fear, an altered metabolism, or all three. There could be flashes of clear reasoning in otherwise confused patients, and movements that were possible one day were not possible the next, but easy again the following week.

My interaction with a wheelchair-bound patient with a brain tumour shows some such phenomena:

At lunch, I assist Mr Merk. Mr Lerner is also there, he can mostly eat alone. Well, not quite: when a plate is standing in front of him, for example, he can only eat things which are on the upper right quarter of the plate. I do not know whether that is due to a problem with movement or with sight. I ask him a couple of times if I should help, but cannot quite make sense of his answers. He refuses to let me pour him his tea – or at least that is my interpretation – but then spills it when pouring it himself. Most of all he continuously tries with his right hand to pull a little table cloth on which a vase with flowers and some other things are standing. I take it away from him a couple of times with the friendly remark that this could go wrong, and with the question whether I could be of any help, and finally I place the cloth completely out of his reach. At that point he gets angry and mumbles something about me being in for a good beating. I do not react to that, but feel a bit hurt. I also feel insecure because in his case I cannot tell at all whether he still reasons clearly [Ger.: klar sein] and just has multiple paralysis, or whether he is totally disoriented.

In all this, biomedical, cultural and psychological causalities became blurred and lost significance for nurses and visitors. While it was taken for granted that physical processes could alter personality, there was also a deep conviction that patients' attitudes and character had a decisive influence on the state of their bodies and especially on the exact time of death, as shall be discussed in chapter five. In nurses' accounts and interpretations of patients, it was often assumed that the development of a patient, in conscious as much as in unconscious people, was due to an interplay of a lot of inextricable factors, be they medical, social, cultural, spiritual or others. The fading away of all aspects of their patients' lives was seen by the nurses as a holistic phenomenon, in which different factors prevailed at different times, in different people, but which they described and reacted to as one continual process.

Up to this point, individual incidents on single days have taken centre stage as the focus of the ethnography. However, in order to give an accurate account not only of isolated incidents, but also of the dynamics of patients' changing situations and nurses' reactions to them, it is necessary to take longer time frames into consideration, to examine how life faded, what patients' illness trajectories had in common and in what ways they were distinct.

Mrs Brunnhofer was about sixty-five years old when she was admitted to the hospice. After a head injury decades earlier she suffered from paralysis of one side of her body and had a speech impediment. She had been diagnosed with progressing cancer some years ago. She maintained a very resolute and good humoured attitude, which some nurses suspected was only a facade covering up a lot of suffering. This psychologising initially put me off, but later I had to admit that there probably was some truth to their judgement. I met Mrs Brunnhofer during my first fieldwork period and, after her death almost a year later, I also interviewed some of her relatives and a volunteer to whom she had felt very close.

When I met her, my first task was to assist with her morning routine and help her decorate her room:

We start with her morning routine. Sit on the edge of the bed with help, stand up with help, turn around with slow, insecure steps, while I pull the net underpants [Ger.: Netzhose] down and remove the incontinence pad [Ger.: Vorlage], then onto the shower chair, then into the bathroom. Take the night gown off there, which is difficult because of the paralysis, push her wheelchair to the wash basin. This all happens quite slowly, and I let Mrs Brunnhofer do whatever she still can do by herself. She takes the tooth paste and opens it with one hand, puts the electric toothbrush into the basin and tooth paste on it, and brushes her teeth while I put the obligatory two dashes of mouthwash into her water glass. Then she takes out her teeth, first the top set, and holds them with her mouth so that I can brush them with the toothbrush at all those spots where she cannot reach. Then the same procedure for the lower prosthesis. Then I wash her, first the face, then the chest. Then the arms – she holds the paralysed one up [with the other] – and then the back and legs. Erika brings a painkiller adhesive [Ger.: Schmerzpflaster]; I take the old one off and stick the new one to Mrs Brunnhofer's back. ... Then I rub her whole body with lotion, put deodorant on her armpits and perfume behind the ears. A clean night-gown, and then I push her wheelchair back into her room and help her to bed. She wants all hospice towels and flannels to be exchanged for her own ones; I comply. During all these procedures we exchange a friendly sentence or two, and step by step she comes up with a list of five things she still wants me to do for her: find her a cardboard box, put her cross up on the wall, water the tulips in the vase, put another pair of shoes beside her bed, and something else. Once she is in bed I open all windows widely, the television is on, it is spring outside. Mrs Brunnhofer is happy, life is so wonderful, she says, simply fantastic. I ask her whether she would not like to come to the kitchen for meals sometimes, she says well, I shall have to on Monday, I say you don't have to do anything here, and I am a bit surprised, well she says, in fact I have sworn to stay in bed until the end of the way.

In this account, Mrs Brunnhofer was still quite mobile; she was interested in her own appearance and the way her room looked, and made her surroundings her own by bringing in her own towels and putting up a cross and pictures on the wall. In spite of her severe illness and the limitations that came with it, it seemed to make her happy that it was spring, that she could put her things in order and that she could count on reliable assistance.

In the weeks after this account, she would be accompanied to church in a wheelchair and receive quite a number of visitors, some from far away places. Sometimes, she wore a wig, and she often gave me detailed orders to look for specific, preferred items of clothing in her wardrobe. There was, however, a first indication of withdrawal: she was not interested in participating in communal meals and meeting other patients, but explicitly insisted she had decided to stay in bed until the end.

Soon after, I also made a note in another diary that I was never sure whether it was only her speech that was limited, or sometimes the thinking behind it, too – typically, I could not quite tell. A week or two later, I noticed that her speech impediment got worse. Again a week or two later, nurses announced at handover that they had made some adjustments to her morning routine, which she had found increasingly exhausting, to make it less stressful. The next note of her which appears in my diaries mentions that it was discussed at handover how she had difficulties with her digestion and excretion, a typical sign of further loss of strength. Then I did not see her for a while, due to a break in my fieldwork and shift arrangements in the hospice, where I primarily worked in other rooms with other patients.

Mrs Brunnhofer has not been in my care [Ger.: jemanden in der Pflege haben] recently, that is, over the whole summer, but I have noticed in passing that she is getting worse, that she cannot stand up by herself anymore, that she cannot go to the toilet without help anymore, and that she recently has not eaten anything apart from ice cream. Her paralysis has also got worse. In fact, I was often in her room in order to bring her the bedpan and assist her with that. Especially her legs have recently troubled her: from the middle of the thigh downwards she reacts to touch with extreme pain. This leads to problems with the bedpan, because she insists that nothing must touch her legs during its use, not even the duvet. She turns over very slowly towards the paralysed side, until her behind comes free and I can slip the bedpan underneath. Then I leave her alone for a couple of minutes, and then she rings the bell and I help her get off the thing. A nurse once pointed out to me how, in spite of her bodily impairment, friendliness and slow speech, Mr Brunnhofer radiates nervousness, which is contagious, and now that I am aware of it I find dealing with her much easier, and calmly check beforehand whether all my working material is there, even when she has already started turning over. Once we are almost done with the procedure when she says something like, it's a real drag, yes I say, it's difficult like this, with all those impediments, well she adds, now one has to bring life to an end this way, and then problems are over, that's how it is, I say, unfortunately they won't go away before, yes she says, not before.

In contrast to earlier diaries, this account shows a lot of change, which came about very slowly, but is more striking here due to the gap in my diaries: Mrs Brunnhofer was at this point confined to her bed and could not go to the bathroom anymore. She also developed pain in her legs which could not be treated and which made urinating routines an ordeal. Her mood was of course affected by this: she became hectic, maybe due to fear of pain, and found her situation increasingly intolerable, as she told me. Her nutrition became limited to ice cream, all else caused her nausea. At this point, Mrs Brunnhofer had lost all interest in her appearance and that of her surroundings. She never wore her wig any more and dressed only in light nightgowns. She continued to lose strength.

Today, Mrs Brunnhofer is not feeling well in the morning. After drinking her chocolate she complains about nausea, and she does not want any lunch, which would have been ice cream. I come to her room at coffee time, she still does not want anything, but then she rings sometime later and Karl says, for sure that is Mrs Brunnhofer who wants her ice cream. She wants the one without the chocolate bits, he says, everything else is fine. He is smoking, so I go and ask, and indeed, she wants ice cream. I tell her how Karl has predicted this, we have a laugh together. I get the ice cream and come back to her room, place it on her stomach and hand her the spoon. I am a little uncertain how to go about this – she is lying horizontally, only able to move one hand, and the spoon is in that hand, so who will hold the ice cream on her stomach? She says nothing, takes the spoon, sticks it into the bowl, cannot scoop anything up, and looks at me. Look, she says, and repeats the sequence. I am confused, and then say, it does not work that way? Spot on, she says kindly, and it dawns on me. I should help you. Yes she says warmly and smiles. I had not been aware that Mrs Brunnhofer was not able to eat by herself any more, so I give her the ice cream, she wants not too much on one spoon, and says she is especially keen on the half-frozen rest.

As I had not seen her regularly for a while again, this next step in the fading of her energy came as a surprise to me: Because of her rapidly decreasing ability to speak, she had to explain to me with gestures that she was not capable any more of lifting the spoon to her mouth, that she needed to be fed. At this point, I also noticed that she often did not remember any more which nurses had been with her in the days or hours before, and she forgot who I was when I had not seen her for more than a couple of days.

When I left the hospice after my second research period, I was sure Mrs Brunnhofer was going to die soon. However, on a visit some months later, the nurses told me that she had lived until a couple of days before. She had continued to eat nothing but ice cream for several months. Her speech had got worse and worse, her thinking more and more confused, and she had become incontinent like most patients in their final days. She had died in the presence of a volunteer with whom she had had a close friendship.

Mrs Brunnhofer, during the time I knew her, turned from a mobile person with interests in her appearance, her surroundings, other people, going to church and the like, into a totally dependent one who could hardly eat, hardly speak and hardly move, and was more and more unable to do the things she had liked to do, or even to execute just the ordinary tasks of her own daily routines. All of this slowly moved beyond her reach, physically and metaphorically speaking. Accordingly, there is some evidence in my material that nursing routines were re-established and renegotiated at several points in this process, due to changes in Mrs Brunnhofer's abilities. Nurses detected such changes and tried to adjust the daily activities of getting up, eating and going to the bathroom to them.

With my account of her, I have tried to illustrate the fading of life which occurred during the illness trajectory of all hospice patients and encompassed all aspects of human existence. Of course, there is no generalisation possible about such trajectories, and I will not attempt to suggest any model. However, most of the changes that went on with Mrs Brunnhofer and could relatively easily be observed in her case because she stayed at the hospice for a relatively long time, would also occur with other patients at one point or another. Thus, as a general phenomenon of fading life, they were the backdrop against which all nursing went on.

Dignity in the Ordinary

Against such a backdrop, hospice care made possible a wide range of behaviours and solutions to patients' problems that would not necessarily have been tolerated in a normal healthcare setting, or for which there would simply not have been enough resources in other institutions. Most patients were very pleased with the treatment in the hospice most of the time, and many were downright enthusiastic.

In the hospice, the subjective well-being and, if possible, enjoyment of the patients was clearly placed above biomedical rules. In fact, it should not be too surprising that once there was no chance for a cure, it became irrelevant whether a given behaviour, for example smoking, was unhealthy or not. The specific outlook of the hospice meant that staff were prepared to acknowledge this situation whenever the patient did, and that staff were prepared to draw clear consequences from it, rather than pretend that there was still hope – or sense – in a biomedical regime, or cover all up in silence. Thus, patients' subjective well-being could be enhanced in many ways.

For one thing, staff saw it as their routine duty not only to help when asked, but gently to facilitate events that would improve patients' subjective well-being. In the following story, told about Hans Dornschuh with whom this book started, two such interventions can be found.

> Hans has visitors today; when I come in there are his ex-wife and two other women. He calls the ex-wife his little mouse, and she also calls herself that. I offer coffee, as I am just doing the coffee round, the mouse accepts, the others at first not, then they change their minds. Hans likes talking about his mouse often and at length, once he says they have become much better friends than before the divorce. Today there is the issue of her possibly sleeping here, Sieglinde has offered that, in case Hans needs support, she says. Both are not sure, Hans seems to think it would be boring for her, and she in turn seems to assume he does not want her, so she goes home and tells Hans, with whom she discusses the issue, she would think it over and call later. Later she calls and comes back to stay.

The first intervention cannot be discerned without some background: at the hospice, it was customary that patients' visitors would be offered coffee and cake, to make their stay nicer and enable patients to be the host in their own rooms – an unusual practice in other healthcare institutions, which surprised many. In this case, the visitors politely refused at first and were then convinced to change their minds.

More significantly, staff encouraged the patient's partner to spend the night in his room. Initially, both the patient and his partner were a bit shy about this offer. Both were not sure whether they might not be a burden for the other. Then, in due time and with the encouragement of at least two members of staff, they changed their minds. The hospice provided a portable bed, sheets and towels.

There seems to be nothing extraordinary as such in helping a patient to smoke as in the account this book started with, offering visitors coffee or sleeping in one's ex-husband's room. Such small accounts are, however, very significant for understanding everyday notions of good nursing at Stadtwald Hospice. In the nurses' daily work, there was no clear boundary between nursing tasks and psychosocial care for patients, between physical and mental wellbeing. They considered taking care of both to be part of their routine. Again, perceptions of hospitals and nursing homes come into play here: When a patient was initially reluctant to use the offers the hospice made beyond routine nursing, or was very shy about asking for something, the nurses often suspected that she had come from a particularly repressive hospital ward.

The Nurses' View – Carers' Interest in Patients' Lives

Such was the situation of the patients – what about the nurses? What were their interests and motivations, what assumptions and values structured their interaction with patients and how were these expressed in daily activities? The next step of the ethnography will turn to nurses' ideas of hospice care and try to show how, even in a setting with a very liberal and caring ethos, there were clear expectations about who patients were, how they ought to live and how their interaction with nurses was to be structured.

Being a Good Girl – Misunderstandings with Mrs Behrens

Mrs Behrens was a woman in her early seventies who, as one nurse put it, 'was down to earth and did not like the cosy ways' of Stadtwald Hospice. She had lung cancer, was very sleepy most of the day and quite grumpy a lot of the time. Apart from that, she could walk, eat and wash herself with hardly any assistance. She spent most of the day dozing in a chair in her room, but did appreciate the company of those who were not deterred by her grumpiness and her black and ironic sense of humour. Once she made a joke about a nurse having given her the wrong injection, which left the nurse, a caring, considerate and slightly naive woman, quite insulted for the rest of the shift. In conversation, Mrs Behrens liked to talk of her pre-war childhood in a region that is now in Poland. She had had a very tough life, with war stories mentioning injury during the war, refugee life, and having to start from scratch afterwards, badly paid jobs all her life, an unfulfilling marriage and estranged children. I had a friendly relationship with her and spent quite some time talking to her and listening to her stories.

The first incident that made me aware that she did not fit the usual hospice treatment of 'patient first' was about medication.

Mrs Behrens takes her medicine today, which she has not done in the last couple of days, for fear of vomiting, she says. She stresses that she is now doing what everybody expects of her, that she is a good girl, and I say, you are not expected to take your medicine, you can decide by yourself.

The incident reveals a misunderstanding about social roles in the hospice. Mrs Behrens probably expected to please me by taking her medicine regularly, but I remained indifferent. By refusing her a traditional patient role (Parsons 1951), in which the patient gains sympathy and acceptance by going along with the biomedical treatment eagerly, I robbed her of a possibility to express herself in such a patient role: She was neither able to voice discontent, sadness or the like by not taking her pills, nor could she express happiness, sympathy or acceptance by taking them – it was all up to her, and she was expected to express herself directly, not indirectly. Mrs Behrens, I conclude, was probably not too interested in such outspoken autonomy concerning her treatment. Maybe, never having been 'in charge' during most of her life, she had had little experience with autonomous decision making in the hospice sense.

A series of little stories about ginger sweets she used to offer me sheds some additional light on the peculiar partiality and limitations of the hospice nursing approach. One day, after a long conversation, Mrs Behrens offered me a piece of candied ginger, which I ate and liked. The next day, when I took some more, she was extremely pleased, but stressed at the same time that the ginger was expensive since it had been organically grown and bought in a special shop. This somehow puzzled me, but I continued to take a piece of candied ginger every now and then when I was in her room. Again some days later, she offered me the whole box as a present, and I was at first quite uncertain how to handle this offer, since, while I liked the ginger, I had eaten some of it just to please her and make her happy.

> She repeatedly offers me candied ginger sweets to take away with me, but finally I leave them here in the room, and say, in the staff room fridge I might forget them, but not here.

The solution I found in the end is quite telling: I accept the present, but leave it in her room rather than take it along to the staff room.

In retrospect, the whole dealings around the ginger sweets explain a lot about our relationship in terms of gifts and exchange, and illustrate the nature of emotions in hospice nursing. It seems to me that Mrs Behrens offered me the ginger in order to make up for all that she was being offered by hospice staff – to offer something herself. That is why she stressed the value of her present, too. When she offered me the whole box, however, and thus extended the exchange beyond the confines of our talk in her room, it became apparent that the offer of friendship and care from my part was limited to certain spaces and to the times of interaction: I ate ginger to please her while in her presence and I was not really interested in more far-reaching exchange of presents beyond the professional friendliness of the nursing relationship. The staff room, the nurses' backstage area, was an area where that relationship did not have the same significance and indeed would probably have been discussed in vaguely therapeutic terms by other nurses and myself. Therefore, I considered it an inappropriate place to keep her present. My friendship with Mrs Behrens had clear limits pertaining to nursing routines and the spatial and emotional organisation of the hospice. Mrs Behrens tried in vain to establish lasting mutuality in her relationship with me. While I was genuinely concerned about her, that concern was subordinate to my role as an eager apprentice nurse.

Such analysis of my experiences with Mrs Behrens sheds a different light on my behaviour towards Mrs Öttinger, where I may at first have appeared quite servile. Ultimately, the power to grant attention, services and friendship – or refuse them – always stayed with the nurses, and their affection was limited to certain times and places. It was from such a power base that extreme patience, friendliness, flexibility and care were enacted and that patients were given the possibility to take charge. In fact, one nurse once said to me that it was easier to adapt even to the most difficult patient knowing that ultimately they would become weak and the nurses would have their way.

Uses of Autonomy – The Nurses' Demands

I have made it clear above that one limitation of the hospice approach became apparent when patients did not appreciate – or understand – the idea of patient-centeredness in the hospice. However, there was also the opposite case – patients who insisted on autonomy, but used it in a different way from what some hospice staff were willing to grant.

> At handover, when the nightshift gets to room number four, Katja begins with the words, well, that's rather bad, and then she tells the usual things: Mrs Hahn does not want to be disturbed, gets along fine, nothing worth mention there. When she has finished Sascha asks, what's bad about that, Katja does not understand, well, what did you mean by 'bad' when you started? Ah yes, we are not allowed to go into the room at night – I just know the patient from hearsay, says Katja. I would not know whether she has blonde or black hair. Or if she is still there at all, says Sven half jokingly, or whether she's that woman who walked out a moment ago. Sascha says OK, we have been having that problem for a couple of nightshifts, and then sighs, half jokingly as well, the control paranoia of our night nurses. Just as well, everybody takes it in a resigned and joking fashion and we move on to the next room, Mr Müller. Already last week, I remember, somebody had asked whether it would be OK if Mrs Hahn lay dead in her room for hours, concerning the exact time of death and all that [for the death certificate].

Mrs Hahn, who is discussed at handover in the diary narrative above, was a patient in her late seventies who was still mobile, could look after herself most of the time and wanted to be alone and do nothing. Her room was bare, she did not pursue any apparent activities, and she did not want to be checked on every hour as was customary at night. All this seemed to disturb some of the hospice staff, and their slight confusion is shown in the passage above. The nurse arguing with the others suggests that this is an issue of control over patients, and the points made are indeed about control. I would, however, argue that there is more to it, namely that many hospice nurses implicitly demanded from patients to get involved with them, to interact and appreciate interaction. It seemed to trouble some nurses when patients who could have interacted refused to do so.

Mr Nolte was a patient in his eighties, a former sociology lecturer who came across as very stern and determined, and as an intellectual. Mr Nolte did indeed claim autonomy, and he did so in ways that the nurses often did not appreciate. He reminded them whenever the medicine was brought late, and he classified staff as 'nursing people', explaining to me that this was a category of people with whom different rules of privacy applied. Mr Nolte had extremely clear ideas about where exactly every little item in his room should be placed, he had brought his own brand of fruit juice, and he wrote down nursing guidelines for his everyday routine. The nurses mainly ignored those guidelines, trying to negotiate these routines with him in conversation instead as was customary.

> I talk to Sieglinde about the orders: Mr Nolte has detailed instructions for his care, a step by step plan for the evening routine for example. Sieglinde rejects that: She does not want to adhere to it because that way she gets the feeling that she is demoted to some sort of servant, who is in a relationship of obedience without a further human factor. It shows to her exactly, she says, 'what Mr Nolte thinks of us'.

There were several further indications of some kind of power struggle between the nurses and Mr Nolte: in his absence, nurses were clearly very anxious not to make even small mistakes in his treatment, which they were not so much with other patients. In his presence, they seemed all the more determined, affectionate and nurse-like, as if to stress the validity of their role and approach. There was a rumour that Mr Nolte had a relationship with a woman several decades younger than himself, who often came to visit. This was told to me with some disapproval by one nurse, which was very unusual for the hospice atmosphere, where normally very few moral judgements were dispensed on all sorts of behaviours sometimes wildly dissident from the societal mainstream.

The tasks and routines completed for Mr Nolte were no different from those done for others. In fact, he was very co-operative and helpful in the actual nursing routines, and he displayed less open fear, anxiety, nervousness and suspicion than some other patients. However, it was precisely this absence of openly displayed emotion that many nurses seemed to find difficult to accept. In conversations amongst themselves they often tried to detect indirect signs of fear and emotional need in his behaviour. The conflict over his notes, and the one nurse's judgement that she was only seen as some kind of servant, both suggest that the acceptance of a personal relationship going beyond the professional level was seen as a precondition for successful work with a patient. Nursing had to be more than a technical procedure, it was to be considered more than merely a service provided by service specialists.

In this respect, the medical gaze in Foucault's sense (1991[1963]) was still present in the hospice. As Armstrong (1984) suggests, it had, however, undergone a transformation from being directed primarily to the patient's physical body, to being concerned with the patient's social, emotional and psychological circumstances. The emotions of the patient were to be unilaterally disclosed, to be examined and discussed. Autonomy, in this view, would be OK only as long as it was based on some trusting disclosure of emotions by the patient, which would give more meaning to nurses' work, too, and which would occasionally transform routine events into narratives of shared relevant life experience.

The decisive aspect of patients' lives to which nurses could make a crucial contribution was positive, or at least meaningful, experience. The professional ambition of most nurses was to help the patients in the remainder of their lives and their pride was to be an important precondition for the patients' well-being at the hospice. Where such a role was not feasible, or even clearly discouraged, as in the case of Mr Nolte, many nurses tended to feel that something was wrong with a patient, or something was missing in their relationship with a patient. These nurses did not only have a certain notion of patients' life at the hospice, they also had an idea of their own role in its construction.

Success and Failure in Hospice Nursing

Success in hospice nursing occasioned many stories. In what follows, I will turn to such success stories and ask what they reveal about hospice attitudes. Further on, I will look at aspects of failure and helplessness again. There were two typical occasions where success stories would be told. One was handover. The other one was when a nurse, after having been in a patient's room, came back to the staff room and reported to those who were sitting there – and since the least qualified people sometimes had the least work, I happened to sit there occasionally and listen to such stories.

'Success' in daily nursing was actively constructed most of the time. Nurses detected a problem, made a plan, and set out to rectify the problem. In doing so, hospice staff were often prepared to go to enormous lengths when they felt that the situation of a patient demanded an unusual or complicated solution, as was illustrated by an event that concerned Hans Dornschuh, who has been mentioned before:

Yesterday it had been extremely difficult to change Hans's incontinence pad. He easily gets out of breath when he gets nervous, is already very weak and loses control of his bladder when he gets excited. That again is extremely embarrassing for him, and makes him all the more nervous, so he gets out of breath even more [Ger.: luftnötig werden], and so on. Today, we go in in a three: Till, Dieter and myself, and Dieter and Till have come up with a new system: while Dieter turns Hans over and holds him up, I put his penis into a urine flask [Ger.: Ente], and Till cleans him and changes the incontinence pad. This way, nothing gets dirty and there is no need for him to be embarrassed. It all works great, Hans stays calm, urinates just a little, which I collect, and in the end we are all very content. He now admits that he had been afraid of the whole affair for some time. His ex-wife is also relieved, and somehow this is one of those moments when staff here are happy about work going well.

In the example, the patient's comfort is ranked quite highly: two nurses spend time working out a plan, three nurses spend considerable time putting it into practice, and all those involved feel quite happy about it afterwards. In contrast, the most efficient biomedical solution could have been not to bother, to ask the doctor to lay a catheter, and there would not have been any comparable work for the nurses with the urine incontinence of this particular patient ever again. It was, however, quite typical that nurses would put a lot of time and energy into finding solutions that made it slightly simpler for patients to keep face and maintain dignity in their often quite distressing situation, and that would delay dependence on biomedical intervention and equipment. When the patients appreciated this, nurses considered their work successful and started to spread the word of their success.

The general pattern displayed in the passage, problem – plan – solution – story, could be encountered frequently at Stadtwald Hospice, if not always in such detailed form:

Judith and Edeltraud have developed a method for Mrs Deimeling to get from her bed to the toilet chair faster and with less exertion. The chair is now at the top of the bed, not at the foot end; she accepts that and is happy.

The careful construction of routines better suited for the patients, enabling them to live with greater comfort and dignity, was one of the nurses' main occasions to talk about the success of their work. Indeed, as shall be discussed in the next chapter, such construction of routines going beyond the normal state of affairs lent itself well to narrativisation, and thus every special solution found enriched not only the patients' life experience but also the nurses' work experience.

While patients' dignity and independence from biomedical solutions were one frequent topic of success stories, another one was pleasant physical experience. Very often a nurse would come into the staff room and say something like 'I helped Mrs X have a bath and she loved it' or 'I massaged Mr Y's shoulders and he was really pleased'.

Once Jürgen and Julia come into the staff room and are apparently very pleased. Mrs Wörner, who is normally very distant, has allowed them to wash her. They seem to have done that very thoroughly and in great detail, and apparently it was pleasant for Mrs Wörner, too. The two of them appear to find this a very harmonious moment. Before, I had had the impression that Mrs Wörner had been much respected, but had allowed no closeness, and that some of the staff had been of the opinion that it would be much nicer for Mrs Wörner to allow at least some.

The passage contains a little story and an indirect commentary I give through adding some of my own impressions and interpretations while writing my diary. The story shows that the nurses take some pride in having persuaded a patient to experience the everyday routine of washing as pleasurable. My own commentary in the diary narrative generalises this into a view that the nurses prefer patients to allow physical and metaphorical closeness.

Pleasant physical experience of everyday routines was thus an important aspect of the life that was sought for patients. However, when analysed with regard to who tells what about whom, the story has a number of further interesting implications. The first one is that there seems to have been a general assumption amongst staff previously that Mrs Wörner did not enjoy being washed. The second assumption is that she did enjoy it at the time in question. There is no direct evidence for any of the two, and still the story made it into the staff room and into my diaries as a success story. Mrs Wörner herself somehow seemed to have only a very indirect voice in declaring her treatment a success.

In this case, the blame could possibly still be placed on a sloppy ethnographer. However, I think there is more to the vagueness of the passage than just bad field-notes. On the one hand, staff interpretations of Mrs Wörner had been inaccurate before – I shall later present an excerpt where a misunderstanding about male nurses caring for her arose. In addition, this story could be contrasted with another account of a patient being washed, this time from a closer perspective:

Dieter [a middle-aged student nurse] has an ostentatiously slow way of washing patients. He explains to Mr Küster that one does not get dirty in bed anyway, but that it is more about refreshing the patient. He hardly uses any soap, announces the tiniest step to the patient beforehand and most of all asks permission every time, which seems strange sometimes with Hans [Dornschuh], who is used to different approaches [from the closed psychiatric ward]. Dieter makes a point of taking a lot of time and doing everything really slowly, Mr Küster once gets quite impatient, I have to smile behind Dieter's back and Mr Küster smiles back. I have the impression that patients are, for Dieter, a kind of meditational object and that some rules, like slowness and great respect, are part of the meditation. I also have the impression that this completely bypasses some patients, who would rather want a jovial style of interaction and a quick end to the tiring procedure of washing.

While in the first passage – with Mrs Wörner – it cannot finally be verified what the patient thought, in the second passage – with Mr Küster – it cannot be proven that the nurse would consider the washing routine a success. However, he definitely did not notice that the patient perceived it as a nuisance. This suggests some caution in taking success stories at face value.

What about failure, though? It struck me in my interviews with nurses that there was a general refusal to talk about failures of the hospice, or even acknowledge the existence of failure. One or more success stories were readily produced by all at even a superficial prompting, but when asked in an interview or daily interaction about 'a time when you felt you could not work with a patient at all, or you failed to deal with a patient's needs', the nurses tended to say that there were, of course, problems, or demanding patients, but the hospice could always adjust and would always adjust. They would then typically mention that one or two patients could not be satisfied at all, but had been extremely rare exceptions in unusually complicated psychosocial circumstances.

The absence of failure is ultimately, as I concluded, a problem of definition, of a term being absent from the nurses vocabulary, a story never told, rather than a sign that all interaction was successful. One solution lies in the temporality of hospice care: in due time, patients would all become weaker. In most cases, that would mean that conflicts would lose intensity, patients would lose energy and be forced to appreciate help more. Ultimately, as one nurse has already been quoted to have said, the nurses would have it their way, a gentle and caring way, but theirs nonetheless. Until that time, and in such context, the liberal patient-centred ethos of the hospice would frame any failed interaction as a problem, a conflict, a mis-understanding – something to be worked on. 'Working on it', however, was already classed as positive, and ultimately the situation would be resolved by the illness trajectory of the patients. Not only were the nurses in a stronger position than the patients in regard to daily routines and medical information, they also knew much better than the patients where the illness would lead them and what ideas and practices most patients would in fact appreciate towards the end.

Notes

1. My analysis here draws inspiration from the work of James Fernandez (1986). Jennifer Hockey (1990), drawing mainly on Lakoff and Johnson (1980), has analysed symbols and metaphors of life and death in a hospice and a nursing home in the northeast of England. Pfeffer (1998) contrasts her work in a hospice with research in a hospital, providing a very useful additional perspective.

2. The image of the household is my own heuristic addition – it was not explicitly present in hospice discourse.

3. In the light of my earlier discussion of late-modern ideas of personhood, it should be empha-sised that the household-related identities mentioned here would of course be quite partial and situational for a given individual, not fully, socially encompassing in all domains of life – at least

not for nurses and visitors. For a critical discussion of the implications of understanding nursing as home work, see for example Ostner and Beck-Gernsheim (1979).

4. Gerstenkorn (2004) has studied German hospice nursing from the point of view of professionalisation theory and gives a more general and detailed picture of nurses' life work seen through interviews. My point here is mainly to provide background information for my own later ethnographic analysis.

5. For very similar considerations on English hospice care see Lawton (1998, 2000).

6. The work of Kübler-Ross (1969) has been much criticised in this respect, as was discussed in chapter one.

4
NURSING STORIES –
NARRATIVE APPROACHES
TO HOSPICE LIFE

Stories in the Negotiation of Hospice Life

In Stadtwald Hospice, the maintenance of professional work standards depended fundamentally on a continuous flow of information between nurses of several shifts, doctors, relatives and other medical personnel. During my fieldwork, I noticed that such information was circulated in two very different forms, which I shall call 'factual information' and 'stories'. Factual information was mainly about the more standardised aspects of nursing, while stories were concerned with the life experience of patients and nurses. Quite early on in my fieldwork, I had the impression that there was a direct relation between the hospice emphasis on lived life and holistic care, and the abundance of stories in Stadtwald Hospice.[1]

Factual information was mostly technical, and it was written down in patients' files after each shift. All matters written down as factual information had financial or administrative implications: the patients had a formal right to certain nursing tasks as part of their treatment, such tasks would appear on the bills of insurance companies, and whether they had been performed could be checked by those government authorities that supervise health institutions. In the patients' files, such information was available to anybody who was authorised to access those files – nurses, administrative staff, doctors and medical authorities. In this form, it was technical knowledge, stripped of the lived experience in which it had once been generated. Pfeffer (1998) rightly points out that there is a close relation between this kind of knowledge and a passive understanding of the patient as subjected to medical control and expertise.

Beyond factual information, however, a different kind of knowledge was passed on and negotiated in Stadtwald Hospice in the form of stories. There were lots of stories about what patients, nurses or relatives had done, of visits received, professional mishaps, interesting conversations, episodes of joy, experiences of helplessness, and so on. I have already told some of them in the previous chapters. Such stories were not part of the patients' files, where normally only a couple of lines would be devoted to the psychosocial aspects of nursing. Stories had no reality for insurance companies or health authorities. Yet, they were the form into which important experiences of patients and nurses were put, through which they became accessible at all, in which they were passed on and in which their meaning was negotiated.

When compared with interviews and statistical surveys – widespread methods in hospice research – the collection of stories has the methodological advantage that they relate to everyday practices rather than prompted abstractions and that they are themselves a constituent of human everyday life. I have already mentioned above that I found interviews with patients of limited value in my research. I did interview some nurses and gained important background information by doing so, but I still argue that the focus on abstract conclusions of expressive people has in the past somewhat distorted the representation of hospices in both the media and research genres. At Stadtwald Hospice, interviews were most easily possible with unusually expressive nurses who were in a sense spokespeople anyway and also had administrative duties related to representing the hospice to the outside. Interviews were thus mostly expert interviews. While this does of course not make them irrelevant in the least, I found it more promising in an inquiry about everyday life and everyday experience to use everyday stories.

My analysis and interpretation of stories is informed by work of the social psychologist Jerome Bruner (1986, 1990), picked up and extended in scope by the anthropologist Michael Carrithers (1991, 1992, 1995, in press) and used successfully in medical anthropology by Cheryl Mattingly (1994, 1998).[2] Stories, in this perspective, are a mode of human thought and repository of human experience. Typically, they are about human endeavours, about people trying to do things and what happened to them as a result. They tell us how a normal state of affairs changed, how this change was dealt with and normality was restored, or how a different normality was established. Thus, stories mediate between the normal and the unusual in human experience, they deal with breaches of the ordinary. In this function, they are deeply relevant both for individual people and social groups.

In relating breaches of the ordinary, stories on the one hand have a normalising function: unusual experience is made accessible for the individual person and the social group, who can then deal with it in some way. On the other hand, stories can also develop subversive powers precisely by framing experiences which are not socially accepted. In addition, they can have unexpected consequences by carrying the author, or the audience, to some conclusion that was never intended in the first place. All of these functions of stories point to a power residing in narrative which is somewhat unpredictable.

There are a number of structural features that define a story: it comprises characters, a narrator and an audience. Within this framework it accounts for events and for the actions, intentions and feelings of the characters in relation to those events. Thus, stories are about the interplay between, on the one hand, events, and, on the other hand, characters – their aims, intentions and inner motivations. Stories relate the events not so much as ordered in mere chronological sequence, but as woven together by causes and effects. The plot of a story, its guiding line of thought, results from such causes and effects – from the way in which the events, the actions and the inner motivations of the characters are causally linked in the light of the narrator's point of view, as interpreted by an audience. Such a plot is the organising principle of a story. It makes it possible to understand the story and to pass it on.

Since the causal relationships in a story are never in any sense 'objective', but always seen in the light of the perception of the characters, the narrator and the audience, the story, its constituent parts and its plot are always open to more than one interpretation. Bruner (1986: 14) distinguishes a landscape of action, which is quite clearly laid out, from a landscape of consciousness, which is less easily accessible. Carrithers (1992: 78) suggests instead talking of an uneven distribution of consciousness between the characters. Different interpretations, tension and surprise result from this uneven distribution. For both the characters and the audience, things can and do turn out differently from what was expected, and in that way the story develops lifelikeness.

Such a story need not be long – if uttered in a meaningful context, one short sentence can suffice to make a 'minimal narrative' (Carrithers 1995: 268). Whether such a textual fragment is a story or not is then dependent on context. Some metaphors, such as the metaphor of the journey so frequently used for our lives and often for 'dying', already necessarily contain a 'story seed' (Carrithers in press) and are meaningful specifically because they call for a plot with which to fill them.

Similarly, it is not always easy to tell what features need to be present to call a text – or a couple of words – a story. Some of the formal criteria given above may at times be present in an implicit form and need to be inferred. However, 'To accept that a story could be evoked rather than told is no more than the corollary of the observation that implicit inference is necessary to all stories' (Carrithers 1995: 268). In what follows, I shall be especially concerned with minimal narratives, which may consist of just a couple of sentences. These need not be looked at exclusively as stories, but interpreting them this way pays attention to how they orient actors in a flow of action, in a dynamic social situation.

One further aspect needs to be mentioned: while it is fruitful for an anthropologist to look at the content of narrative, attention must also be paid to its social function. There is always an interplay between content and function of a story, and the telling can become a significant social performance in itself. Stories do, on the one hand, reveal events, attitudes and actions, but they are, on the other hand, instrumental in establishing, directing and negotiating them.

In this way, they do not just look to the past, but also to the future. Narratives, as Byron Good writes, 'not only report and recount experiences or events, describing them from the limited and positioned perspective of the present. They also project our activities and experiences into the future, organising our desires and strategies teleologically, directing them toward imagined ends or forms of experience which our lives or particular activities are intended to fulfil' (Good 1994: 139). They do so in individual minds, but also in the social context in which they are told.

In Stadtwald Hospice, accordingly, stories were not just about the psychosocial life of hospice patients, they also had a lot to do with how that life was perceived and organised by the nurses. Stories had a legitimating function for the behaviour of nurses in the past and served as behavioural suggestions for the future at the same time. They had a programmatic aspect, and by saying what happened and how, it often followed from them how a nurse should interact with a certain patient in the future. Stories provided moral guidelines, 'aesthetic standards' (Carrithers 1992: 63–66) of nursing behaviour.

Such stories went through ever changing perspectives. When I write of the function of stories, I do not mean to say that the function of one given story was the same for everybody, or even for any two people, or that no other form of communication could have the same function. Similarly, not everybody was equally involved in the telling and circulation of stories. There were staff and patients who talked a lot, openly and with pleasure. Others told only few stories, and most were selective in what was told to whom and when. There seemed to be a general tendency for experienced and highly qualified staff to tell less stories, especially at handover, while inexperienced staff talked the most, and novices kept quiet. However, when experienced staff did tell stories, their stories were usually much more dramatic, authoritative and emotional. Possibly less experienced staff needed more reassurance through their stories, while more experienced staff set more compelling behavioural suggestions through theirs.

Toni Schultz, one of the most demanding patients the hospice had during my fieldwork time, provides an example of how stories provide guidance and legitimation in the daily organisation of hospice care.

Mr Schultz, whom we all call Toni, has been a traveller, fifteen years in Asia, somebody says. He is around fifty years old. His room is full to the brim with all sorts of Buddhist and Hindu devotional items, statues, pictures of yogis, incense sticks and hand-written notices about the power of love and similar themes. There are also a couple of photographs of him, from a time when he was already ill, but still looking joyful, quite a handsome man with a cunning expression on his face and a marked nose. Toni is not so well now, he has lost a lot of weight, is confined to bed and complains of pain in all sorts of places. He smokes joints, which his friends roll for him, the room always smells strongly of hash and incense. The Tibetan Book of The Dead in an edition by Sogyal Rimpoche and a standard book by Kübler-Ross are in the room.[3]

Toni is considered very difficult; apparently he has lots of special wishes, while it is impossible to do anything right for him. He also has very precise ideas about his medication, which of it to take when and which not at all, and he takes a whole lot of Steiner stuff [Ger.: 'Anthromedis', nursing slang for anthroposophical medicine] and massages with anthroposophical oils. He continues to complain about pain, in the legs most of all, but refuses most pain killers and wants to master the pain by changing positions and supporting himself with cushions [Ger.: Lagerung]. Once I come into the room to change the sheets and we discover, one by one in different corners of the room, scores of cushions for that purpose. As mostly with such patients, the team [Ger.: 'das Team'; nursing staff] seems to agree that great fear is at the base of his sensitivity to pain and his continuous demands. Within the team it is contested whether he has any physical pain at all.

Already in this first description of Toni, some themes from former sections of this study occur again: he had unusual freedom in decorating his room lavishly, smoking cannabis, refusing medication, using alternative medication and having lots of friends around a lot of the time. There are also again hints towards typical nursing attitudes: Alongside the observation that he is difficult and demanding, I write that he 'has lots of special wishes while it is impossible to do anything right for him'. From my nursing perspective, I seem to have found it difficult to accept that he made staff work without being thankful or having clear aims; in short, that he did not appreciate all that hospice care offered. I wrote down a similar remark by one of my colleagues at handover:

> On one of these days, Klaus says that he now tells himself, every time he goes into the room, there is nothing you can do for him, when you leave here he will be as unhappy as before.

The most difficult type of patient behaviour seemed to be when a patient's wishes could not be satisfied, or when a patient made demands which were, for whatever reason, not meant to be satisfied.

Over a period of several weeks, dealings with Toni proved to be extremely demanding for staff and were seen as problematic by almost all of the nurses. In order to illustrate my overarching point of stories as behavioural suggestions, I will first consider a short narrative that was told at handover:

> At handover, there is prolonged talk about Toni. Matthias was on the nightshift and says, whenever Toni heard him, even from far away on the corridor, he started to cry and to moan but then had no concrete problem with which he could help. Finally, Matthias says, he ignored him at times and just had a careful look later, to see it was nothing urgent. Christa says that she now immediately asks Toni for the order of priority of his requests, and everything which he does not bring up after one or two ques-

tions she considers not so important. Otherwise, he would always find a new job at the end of the previous one.

This passage contains a small story about Toni and Matthias, followed by the comment of another experienced nurse. I would argue that the story of Matthias and Toni has mainly rhetorical character. It legitimates – to himself and to his colleagues – Matthias' decision to ignore the patient at times. It also functions as a possible guideline by suggesting that this behaviour has already proven to be adequate and could continue to be used by others in the future. The other nurse, in fact, immediately takes this implicit suggestion up and tells a minimal story about her own technique she uses to leave the patient limited scope in expressing lots of wishes. She thus supports Matthias' opinion that Toni's wishes are largely pointless and that a minimising strategy has to be developed in order to tackle this problem. We are dealing with an implicit, minimal negotiation on how to handle Toni.

Stories are, in Bruner's (1986: 24–26) sense, 'underdetermined'. In our context, they may legitimate past behaviour and suggest future behaviour, but they do not justify a certain behaviour in detail, or put down a concrete, binding rule. Neither do they necessarily mention that legitimation or guidance for the future are at stake at all. Their function is much more subtle, in that they leave scope for interpretation, for agreement or disagreement, which makes them a form especially viable for negotiating social practice. It is significant that the nurse does not say: 'he is not genuine, I have decided to ignore him and I suggest you do the same'. Rather, Matthias tells a small story, comprising attitudes and events, organised by a plot, in order to say much the same thing in a crucially different way.

The importance of stories for legitimation and guidance is underscored by the way they were circulated and, indeed, meant for circulation. A story which was considered significant by a number of nurses at handover would often be told again at least until the same shift came back to work the next day. That means it was told in two further handovers. It could then be assumed that most nurses working that week would know it. In the days after, the story would be mentioned in an abbreviated form only, and just the measure that was taken as a consequence would be told ('There was that incident with Toni's friends and we decided to …'). However, the brief mention indicated that there was a story and made it possible to ask if necessary. In this way, nurses coming back to work after their days off could question the whole story. They would recall it by asking about the abbreviation ('What exactly happened with Toni's friends?') Then they could accept the story, doubt it, reinterpret it or contrast it with another.

One hospice patient, Mrs Wörner, who has been mentioned in the previous chapter, was not very appreciative of the affectionate ways of the hospice nurses. One male nurse once told a story of how he had washed her and had had the clear impression that she did not want to be washed by a man. This was accepted as a matter of fact and the consequence was that, for several days, the patient was only looked after by female nurses, with the remark at handover that she did not like to be in close contact with men. After some time, a new story questioned this:

> Micha tells us how Mrs Wörner had greeted him with the words 'Finally, somebody sensible today' – not exactly charming for all those who had been in the room before him. He concludes that it is not true that she generally does not want to be looked after by men. We talk about this briefly, whether there is maybe an oversensitivity of the hospice in such matters, but we reach no conclusion. Micha says, however, that what has been said once at handover develops a dynamic all by itself and can hardly be undone afterwards, and that is also certainly true in my opinion.

After this, the patient was again looked after by men without any problems, the old story had been overruled as a guideline. The passage shows that there was a clear awareness amongst nurses of the power that stories told at handover had in the organisation of daily hospice routines.

Stories did not only figure prominently in the organisation of nurses' behaviour towards patients, but also in their dealings with other people at Stadtwald Hospice. I have written down an episode, again related to Toni Schultz, where two nurses tell stories about how they dealt with Toni's numerous visitors:

> Already, on the day before, Ludwig had said that there were so many people in the room that one had to ask for permission to pass through when going about one's daily work. Then, he says, while laying a new butterfly [a type of infusion needle] everybody [all of these visitors] kept staring at his hands, and Toni's life partner got excited. It's impossible, she said, doing this [replacing the needle] three times in two days. He just replied, it can even be necessary ten times in one day, when the tissue is like it is in his case. Having finished with the needle, he then told her triumphantly how he had in fact never laid this type of needle before, how nice it was that it still had worked out all right. Later in the day, Horst removed scores of empty water bottles from the room and said, any complaints to be directed to him, but it was impossible to work in a room with so much stuff standing around.

At face value both stories, told to me in the staff room, relate how nurses felt that Toni's many confident visitors were encroaching upon their professional space, and how they made it a point to demonstrate that they would not be intimidated or yield, but pursue their professional life as usual. Of course, on a second level of interpretation, when viewed in the context of their telling, the stories show something slightly different: The nurses felt a need to defend their space and they also felt a need to tell their colleagues about their small victories, thereby suggesting, not without a sense of humour, that resistance was possible and had been put up.

On a third analytical plane, the stories are excerpts from a negotiation that went on between the patient and his visitors on the one hand, who were trying to exercise their hospice right to organise Toni's life in a patient-centred way, and the nurses, who had certain minimal requirements for actual and metaphorical space to work in, on the other. Even in patient-centred nursing, not everything is negotiable. In any case, the stories had the double function of legitimation for actors' own actions and of behavioural suggestion for others.

The question remains, of course, as to why hospice nurses should at all resort to such quite indirect techniques of negotiating daily procedures and establishing institutional standards in psychosocial matters. In other healthcare contexts, it would have been quite feasible for the first nurse in the last example to insist that everybody leave the room while medical treatment was taking place, and the second nurse could just have established a rule for no more than three bottles to be in the room at a given time.

I suggest that this did not happen mainly because an indirect approach fits the emphasis on patient-centred, holistic nursing in a self-reflexive context much better than the explicit establishment of binding, possibly written, rules. At least when it comes to psychosocial matters in a hospice context, any rule would be temporary anyway, as it would have to be based on the nurses' renewed experience and interpretation of a given patient's changing behaviour and mood. In fact, in the highly self-reflexive atmosphere I have described in chapter two, most nurses would be aware that their own interpretation of such patient behaviour was individual and subject to revision – that there was no legitimating biomedical objectivity when it came to holistic care. Thus, an indirect communication strategy, suggesting standards for dealing with patients and relatives without fixing them too rigidly, allowed for the leeway the social configuration of Stadtwald Hospice needed in order to accord with hospice values.

An indirect style of negotiating standards, mediated through use of stories, often drawn out over a period of several days, with continuous and renewed reassurance by double checking one's position with colleagues and patients, seemed to be a pervasive style of communication at Stadtwald Hospice. One more advantage of this style – for both patients and nurses – was that in conflicts loss of face on any side was avoided, that decisions, once they were taken, mostly had strong majorities amongst staff and were usually grounded in careful observation of patients' changing behaviour, while some leeway for personal interpretation remained. Of course, this style also had drawbacks, often ambiguities persisted and consensus could take a lot of time and energy to emerge. An outside doctor once told me that he was sceptical of the frequent changes in the treatment of some patients at the hospice, which depended on the personal styles of the nurses in charge.[4]

Patients thus could rely on a lot of flexibility and openness when dealing with staff and maximum attention would be paid to their individual psychosocial situation over a period of time. Most patients immediately appreciated this. However, sometimes patients who were not used to such an atmosphere seemed to be left with a certain lack of orientation, and at other times negotiations with very demanding patients brought staff to the limits of their energy.

Mr Urban was a man in his eighties who was at the time extremely weak and confined to bed, but fully conscious and clearly aware of everything around him. Most nurses considered him a very difficult patient. The following discussion of his example draws on the above findings about narrative as a currency for social negotiation, but also extends the analysis to the question as to what kind of life it was that was negotiated.

> Since handover, Mr Urban has been on the agenda. He has a broken arm and a healthy one. It is out of the question for him to move the broken arm, but in the last couple of days he has also refused to move the healthy one, saying that it caused him pain. **[A]** Edeltraud [an experienced nurse] explains at handover, at great length, how she caught him scratching his face with the supposedly immovable arm, and how she has introduced a training goal, namely to teach him at least to drink by himself. She explains all this in detail and is proud of her gifts of observation and her stern manner – at least so it seems to me. It is about preserving quality of life for him, she says, because it cannot be that he lies in bed all day thinking about what he cannot do: he should rather concentrate on what he is still able to do. **[B]** In the course of the day there are more stories about Mr Urban: apparently he had a clock put up for him in his room, and, as I remember now, he always had an alarm clock on his bed covers before he got the clock. However, he now seems to keep staff busy by making them check whether the clock is right, whether the hand for the seconds is moving OK, and the like. Edeltraud has apparently already threatened to take the clock down again. **[C]** Now I also remember that Mr Urban started, shortly after having been admitted, to pay extreme attention to whether he got a urine bottle with a short or a long neck. He wanted a short one, the difference seemed minimal to me. **[D]** With Mr Urban, as Bruno [a civilian service worker] states today, one is sometimes forced to talk plainly [Ger.: *Klartext reden*]: he has told him that it is not acceptable to look around the room searching for new ways to keep staff busy while he, Bruno, is still busy with his previous request. Mr Urban should tell him everything that needed to be done, right at the beginning, and then he would do that, and that would be it.

The passage consists of a number of smaller narratives, from which a larger one is built. It shows how ways of living are negotiated which are aligned to ideas and practices in the hospice. The overarching diary narrative begins by mentioning that all these stories about Mr Urban started at handover, and then it goes on to give some background information about him. Within the passage as a whole, there is then a first story, told originally by an experienced nurse at handover:

> **[A]** Edeltraud [an experienced nurse] explains at handover, at great length, how she has caught him scratching his face with the supposedly immovable arm, and how she has introduced a training goal, namely to teach him at least to drink by himself. She explains all this in detail and is proud of her gifts of observation and her stern manner – at least so it seems to me. It is about preserving quality of life for him, she says, because it cannot be that he lies in bed all day thinking about what he cannot do: he should rather concentrate on what he is still able to do.

The nurse had spotted some incongruent behaviours of Mr Urban – he was apparently, in a limited way, stronger and more mobile than he admitted, or realised. She seemed to assume that making such observation was an important part of her work – she was proud of it. She also immediately reacted by introducing a kind of therapeutic target: the patient should learn how to drink by himself. There is a strong implication that independent drinking was a normative target that may require overcoming some resistance from the patient himself. It is not mentioned in the diary that Mr Urban in fact received a special cup with a special straw for all this.

The development of the passage indicates that the nurses continually told each other stories about Mr Urban during the whole shift. The next one, about his clock, is concerned with the amount of work Mr Urban causes:

[B] In the course of the day there are more stories about Mr Urban: apparently he had a clock put up for him in his room, and, as I remember now, he always had an alarm clock on his bed covers before he got the clock. However, he now seems to keep staff busy by making them check whether the clock is right, whether the hand for the seconds is moving OK, and the like. Edeltraud has apparently already threatened to take the clock down again.

It is not clear who tells this small story – grammatical markers indicate that it consists of some things I had heard and some things I had experienced myself. The story makes the point that Mr Urban was a difficult patient who wanted to get additional attention by finding all sorts of reasons to keep the nurses busy in his room. The same nurse who had made it her goal to educate him towards more independent behaviour threatened to remove the clock he seemed to use as a pretext.

The topic of unnecessary amounts of work is taken up in the next story, which I told to myself in my diary, remembering how I had had a lot of work fulfilling Mr Urban's wishes:

[C] Now I also remember that Mr Urban started, shortly after having been admitted, to pay extreme attention to whether he got a urine bottle with a short or a long neck. He wanted a short one: the difference seemed minimal to me.

In the final story, a colleague doing civilian service in the hospice tells me about a conversation he had had with Mr Urban. This story serves as a kind of summary to the former three:

[D] With Mr Urban, as Bruno [a civilian service worker] states today, one is sometimes forced to talk plainly [Ger.: Klartext reden]: he has told him that it is not acceptable to look around the room searching for new ways to keep staff busy while he, Bruno, is still busy with his previous request. Mr Urban should tell him everything that needed to be done, right in the beginning, and then he would do that, and that would be it.

Here, my colleague tells me how he pointed out to Mr Urban that he was demanding too much from staff and that this needed to be rectified. In doing so, he makes explicit what had been mainly implicit before, and thus he takes the negotiation to a more categorical level, resulting in a behavioural guideline.

These four stories appear in my diary in a very condensed form. In the story about the clock, it is not exactly clear who is the original narrator. In my own story about the urine bottle, I do not mention that I had to go back and forth between Mr Urban's room and the equipment room several times to fetch different models for him to try out.[5] In the final story, Mr Urban himself is only implicitly present as an actor.

However, all four still meet the criteria for a story set out before: They all tell about departures from nursing normality. More precisely, they present a process of negotiation between staff and Mr Urban about what is normal and acceptable in looking after him, and how he ought to behave and organise his life. They all tell about characters, their intentions and their actions, and present different points of view on the events. In fact, they thus make up a fifth story, told in my diary, which uses the four smaller stories to account for the whole negotiation process. In this fifth, overarching story, members of staff on the one hand negotiate with Mr Urban. On the other hand, they reassure themselves about a common course of action by exchanging their stories about him. In this way, they make sure that their actions are in line with one another and that a common point of view can be achieved. This common point of view appears in the fourth, more categorical story, where it is made explicit to Mr Urban himself and translated into a clear – if maybe preliminary – guideline for further interaction.

I myself as a member of staff took part in the whole process of negotiation and mutual reassurance. The presentation of it is of course through my own perspective, through my own diary narrative. There, several other perspectives are summarised in the story the anthropologist tells to himself and later to his readership. However, the fact that it was my colleague who had the last, categorical word in it strongly suggests that the process I analysed here was more than just my own, individual process.

The whole episode once again stresses the importance of self-reliance as a value in hospice nursing. In addition to that, the stories about Mr Urban also reveal some more nurses' attitudes towards the patient's life: it is stressed that obstacles need to be overcome through continuous effort, based on the exploration and acceptance of one's own limitations. Self-reliance thus seems to be the base for a kind of self-training ethics, for giving one's best in facing up to the inevitable, progressing illness, and for making the most out of fading life.

Furthermore, the passage supports the view that a lot of what the hospice had on offer depended on the patient agreeing that he was put in charge of his own life, and being willing to make the most of his situation. Once he accepted this, staff were willing to go out of their way to help. They did, however, have difficulties accepting a style of patient behaviour which abandoned conscious control, but remained demanding nonetheless. As one very enthusiastic volunteer at Stadtwald Hospice once put it to me in an interview, 'of course some patients have never had responsibility for their own lives, but then it is our duty to make them accept that responsibility'.

This does not mean that patients were not allowed to abandon hope – they were. Patients' decisions to give up, or to retreat into themselves, were normally respected. At the most, they were approached using the more subtle methods of therapeutic emplotment analysed below. However, patients who made explicit, high demands on nurses were, in my research experience, required either to take charge of their lives, or to remain passive altogether.

On a very practical plane, when patients set themselves conscious goals in daily life, that also made it much easier for the nurses to give them all kinds of support. Setting conscious goals was therefore encouraged, while making demands without a clear direction was discouraged. From the nurses' point of view, self-reliance and self-training did not necessarily imply that patients make grand decisions, plan large independent undertakings or ponder deeply about the meaning of life. Rather, it meant that patients were expected to express their desires about everyday affairs in a way that made it possible for the nurses to respond to them, and that they took on all tasks they could do themselves without help. Thus, an emphasis on self-reliance not only had implications for the patient, but also involved nurses' desires as to how they liked to run their professional lives.

The Meaning of Small Things – Therapeutic Emplotment in Hospice Nursing

Up to this point, the analysis has focused on narrative accounts of everyday practices as pointers for underlying values and attitudes at Stadtwald Hospice. The following section will take a slightly different angle and look at the same issues through an analysis not of finished stories told by a single narrator, but of narratives in the making, constructed through interaction. I will show that hospice nursing very often displayed quite distinct and repeating patterns of both action and communication, namely patterns that Cheryl Mattingly (1994, 1998) has described as 'therapeutic emplotment'. Therapeutic emplotment was frequently used in hospice nursing to establish meaningful experience for patients against the backdrop of steadily fading life.

In her ethnographic study of occupational therapists and their patients in a spinal chord unit in the U.S., Mattingly (1998) shows how patients and therapists often engage in the creation and negotiation of a shared plot structure, guiding their actions through time by placing them in a larger, yet unfinished story which is projected into the future. In turn, the vision of that future gives meaning to the individual actions and experiences within the plot structure. Mattingly shows how occupational therapists, in minute daily interactions such as helping a severely disabled patient to comb his hair, create a goal for the patient, such as looking good when he meets his family. This goal is then used to motivate the patient for further therapy. Mattingly refers to the resulting creation and negotiation of a shared plot as therapeutic emplotment: 'healers actively struggle to shape therapeutic events into a coherent form organised by a plot' (1994: 811). The operation is called emplotment because a desirable narrative figure, a plot, a small story, is suggested from the beginning as the outcome of the interaction: the therapist came; I learned to comb my hair again; now I can look good when I meet my family. The actual realisation of that shared story is then worked towards in further therapy. In all this, however, it is not the emplotted story itself that has the greatest significance. Mattingly argues that the purpose of therapeutic emplotment is the creation of desire (1998: 107) leading towards significant experience (1998: 154f). In occupational therapy as well as in hospice nursing, these two notions are the guiding categories for therapeutic emplotment.

Mattingly's notion of therapeutic emplotment rests on one basic claim: 'We make as well as tell stories of our lives and this is of fundamental importance in the clinical world. Narrative plays a central role in clinical work not only as a retrospective account of past events but as a form healers and patients actively seek to impose upon clinical time' (1994: 811). Mattingly extends the application of terminology generated in narrative analysis to the realm of action, saying that not only past stories, but also actions in the present and plans for the future are governed by narrative structures. With Paul Ricoeur (1981) she argues that action is closely related to narrative.

In order to locate experience in therapeutic emplotment, Mattingly presents her concept as a particular way of structuring time, especially the experience of passing time. The emplotment of chronological time into narrative time facilitates change and meaningful experience and feeds desire for further change and experience. According to Mattingly (1994: 813–14; 1998: 84–85), narrative time thus created has six important features:

(1) It is *configured*, meaning that the structure governed by the plot is a distinct whole.
(2) It is *structured by action and motive*, i.e. created through individual actions of characters with individual motivation.
(3) It is *organised in a gap* between present state and aspirations.
(4) It shows *change*, in fact mostly unexpected change.
(5) It is *dramatic* through the presence of conflicts and obstacles.
(6) The *outcome of things* is *uncertain*.

In her ethnography, Mattingly shows convincingly how all these criteria can be applied to therapeutic interaction, which is fuelled by the desires of the therapist and the patient (2) and aims at a story, not only to tell, but to have been part of, to have experienced in therapy (1). It tries to overcome obstacles (5) on the way to a better future for the patient (3), hopefully transforming her abilities and experience (4), but never certain if, how and when this end can be achieved (6).

Before all this can happen, however, the desire of the patient to engage in therapy at all has to be kindled. Mattingly convincingly shows in great detail how occupational therapists kindle patients' desire for change in minute daily routines, even just through movement alone, and thus subtly seduce them to join in their therapeutic efforts and start emplotting clinical time to make narrative, therapeutic time.

It was a subtle seduction to experience and to plan which I seemed to observe in hospice nurses' approaches towards patients as well and which first led me to consider the application of Mattingly's ideas in the hospice context, an idea that turned out to be quite productive. There is one theoretical issue, however, in which I disagree with Mattingly. She makes it a central focus of her book to argue that there is a homology between narrative and experience, that narrative and experience, because they share the same structure, are of the same kind (Mattingly 1998: 84f, 154f). I suspect that there is a terminological problem here, namely 'action' and 'experience' are used as interchangeable categories, which I personally believe they are not. There is convincing evidence in Mattingly's research that the structures of action and narrative are organised in a similar manner. My own ethnography contributes to this finding. However, I do not see a homology between narrative and experience, because experience – seen here as the moment in all its qualities as they simultaneously appear to an individual human being – can never be adequately captured in narrative. In my own ethnography, I do not claim to be able directly to capture the experience of others, let alone cancer patients whose experience of their life world I can hardly imagine. Even though good stories may be the closest we can get to the experience of others, the boundaries between stories told and the actual experience actors have remains, in my view, insurmountable.

There are also a number of crucial ethnographic differences between the hospice scenario and the occupational therapy scenario studied by Mattingly. In occupational therapy, the desire of patients is directed towards a better future. The time scale, in many ways, is longer than in hospices – if a spinal chord patient decides to engage in therapy, training, in one form or another, might go on for the whole remaining time of his life. Also, while the outcome of therapy is never certain, it is quite likely that an improvement once made will last, a skill learned will be executed regularly. The likelihood of lasting improvement seems to be a crucial factor kindling desire and motivation, making therapeutic emplotment possible.

In the hospice, however, a lot of time is not available, and deteriorating health may mean that any improvement made might be put into doubt again the next day by the physical and mental changes the illness causes. The introduction of the process of fading life has shown that room for targeting desire and directing hope is very limited and that all improvement will certainly be futile in a not-so-distant future. So the question of which goal patients' desire can be directed towards, which kind of experience is to be facilitated and which final story therapeutic emplotment can aim at demands an answer much different from the one given in an occupational therapy context.

In what follows, I will locate therapeutic emplotment in the context of Stadt-wald Hospice. In doing so, the aim of the discussion is not so much to prove or disprove whether emplotment in Mattingly's sense happened, how often, and how accurately. I would like to present emplotment as an important attitude and practice of hospice nursing, sometimes almost hidden, sometimes strikingly evident, but always pliable and underdetermined in the sense stories are, not as a strictly patterned cultural or behavioural script. In sticking with my aim to provide a comprehensive ethnography of hospice nursing at the same time, I have structured the discussion around some important work areas of basic nursing, namely food and drink, mobility, and the facilitation of social contacts.

Breakfast for Mr Tanner

Together with hygiene-related practices, assisting patients with eating and drinking was probably the most important task of hospice nursing. It was an area where the emplotment of small routines into larger structures, facilitating significant experience, struck me most. I will discuss a longer diary excerpt here, related to Mr Tanner. He was a patient in his late forties who stayed at the hospice for many months, suffering from a brain tumour. His torso and legs had stiffened and were mostly immobile. He could not speak well any more and when he did so, he talked in staccato bursts. A lot of the time he would seem absent, typically fiddling with the handrail of his bed or anything else that was in his reach.

> The day starts with breakfast for Mr Tanner. At first, he says he does not want anything, but when I go to the kitchen and tell them, they tell me to ask again – there are boiled eggs on Sundays, you know. Immediately and loudly, Mrs Werner also says yes, Mr Tanner likes a boiled egg, and I remember that he enjoyed his fried eggs with roast potatoes for lunch yesterday very much. So I go back to him and ask, and in fact, he wants a boiled egg. That I give him, always a spoonful of egg with a bite of bread.

There was a documentation file in the kitchen recording what patients had eaten, when and how much; kitchen staff were informed about a lot of patients' personal likes and dislikes regarding food. There were arrangements in place for remembering and providing what Mr Tanner liked – in this case, eggs. His initial refusal to eat was a point where I could just have started on my next tasks – if this was his will, why not let him have it? After all I did not know whether he was maybe feeling nauseous, or simply not hungry. However, when I related my finding back to the kitchen, ready to take on a new assignment, the staff there were not happy with it. They wanted something more for Mr Tanner, namely that he enjoyed what they knew he normally enjoyed. He was to be lured out of his indifference, and so I was sent back with the offer to make him eggs, which he accepted.

> Then I ask him whether he maybe also wants a jam sandwich, yes he says, I order one in the kitchen, come back, he says he would prefer white cheese on it [instead of butter]. I go back to the kitchen again; everything is already prepared: a plate with four small jam sandwiches, each one with a different sort of jam, and there is white cheese on them all, his wishes are already known.

Mr Tanner's appetite had been kindled by the first offer, and kitchen staff were more than ready to go on with providing his favourite foods, carefully prepared, even ahead of his own request and slightly more elaborate than had been asked for. All this was in striking contrast to my own nursing home experience, where feeding had often been little more than the intake of nutrients.

> In the end he eats only one of the sandwiches, I ask him whether he would like a smoke; he says yes. I light him one and stay there – it would be dangerous to let him smoke by himself, as he does not see well at all, and is quite uncoordinated because of his brain tumour, all movements have a strong tilt to the right. I have to remind him to knock the ashes off every now and then. During the course of the week he once had burns on his finger, it seems that he does not have enough feeling left in the hand in question to notice the heat on time. He inhales very deeply and enjoys it very much, the cigarette glows strongly and burns down almost to the filter. We talk a little; I talk more, because he can only talk in short, staccato sentences. It is about smoking habits, I tell him about mine. In between Erika comes in and tells me to join him and smoke, I say no, I just told Mr Tanner I only smoke when I am at a party. He says smoking is the only thing that is left for him, I ask whether he likes a beer every now and then, he says no, he would forbid himself that. I remember now that he used to have an alcohol problem. ... I ask whether his wife was going to come in again today, he says yes, probably, I ask what she does, she is a secretary. The cigarette is finished: he has some trouble putting it out, I have the impression that he has to keep repeating the same movement, unable to interrupt, a kind of feedback loop, many small pressing movements into the ashtray. After a while I take the cigarette away from him and put it out myself.

After breakfast, at my prompting, it was smoking time. A lot of interrelated signs of fading life discussed in the first section of this chapter are present here: Mr Tanner had limited control over his movement and speech, and I only deduced from outer evidence that he did not feel his one hand anymore, something I could not be quite certain about. However, with my help, Mr Tanner enjoyed smoking; it was hardly a coincidence that the conversation turned to that topic as well. Another nurse prompted me to join in and smoke a cigarette myself – clearly trying to teach me a professional nursing gesture to affirm my solidarity and company, more for therapeutic reasons than for my own enjoyment.

The seemingly banal story of Mr Tanner's breakfast illustrates the notion of therapeutic emplotment well when considered as a whole. Attention must be paid to the starting point of the narrative and to its final form: at first, I asked if he wanted to eat, he said no, and I could have left. There would have been no story whatsoever. The final result of the interaction, however, was strikingly different: Mr Tanner had a satisfying breakfast of his favourite foods, he smoked a cigarette and engaged in some conversation with me about smoking and about his wife. If we had been asked about what we did that morning, both Mr Tanner and myself would have had something to tell. In fact I told my diary – an indication that something had happened to which I attributed some importance beyond the normal routines of helping a patient to eat.

Therapeutic emplotment is what happened in between the initial prompting to eat and the story finally told: a shared plot line evolved at the repeated suggestive prompting of staff, telling Mr Tanner that there was more to his morning than he assumed: tasty eggs, different kinds of jam, a cigarette. Right from the start, staff aimed at a story which would somehow include a pleasant eating experience for Mr Tanner. In fact, this unravelled in due course: he voluntarily went along with their suggestion and in the process started voicing some of his own wishes, such as white cheese instead of butter. His desire was kindled and channelled by staff into experiencing Sunday breakfast as a pleasant and meaningful activity. He was, however, not the only beneficiary: staff ended up with a satisfying story to tell about how Mr Tanner did not want to eat on Sunday morning but had such a great breakfast in the end – a kind of story some of the nurses would have told with great satisfaction at handover.

If the success of an emplotment strategy, transforming chronological time into narrative time and changing passing events into meaningful experience, can be measured by the application of Mattingly's six criteria for narrative time discussed above, successful emplotment had gone on: we do end up with a configured narrative, governed by action and motive, showing change situated in a gap between present state and aspirations. In the beginning, the ending of the whole episode was yet uncertain, Mr Tanner's cooperation still had to be ensured. The only feature less obvious is drama: we encountered no spectacular obstacles and conflicts on our way; they were rather located in the help and assistance itself that the episode was about. In all, there is no doubt that chronological, linear time, which just passes, was transformed into narrative time, in which something significant happens.

I have also chosen this story as the first one in a series because there are hints at my own training in strategies for kindling desire and emplotting daily activities: initially, I was prepared to break off the interaction, but kitchen staff kept it going. Later, the nurses tried to make me engage further with Mr Tanner by lighting my own cigarette, encouraging me to switch from an assisting to a participatory attitude in my nursing practice. In the later course of my fieldwork, I would attempt to create interactive stories like that of Mr Tanner's breakfast by myself, if not always successfully, as will be shown below.

There is, in addition, one last point that has to be noted concerning Mr Tanner's breakfast, again relating to the nurses' perspective as found in my diary narrative: there is a clear indication here that meaningful experience was created, not just for Mr Tanner, but also for myself, the nurse. I would suggest that this is what made the emplotment perspective, and maybe work in the hospice as such, attractive for staff: the emphasis at Stadtwald Hospice was on the ever changing situations of individual patients, creating diverse and challenging experiences for nurses, rather than on the strict adherence to routine procedures that characterises most hospitals and nursing homes.

Cheryl Mattingly stresses that attempts at emplotment are always uncertain and that obstacles and conflicts are part of the process (Mattingly 1998, esp. 96–97, 129–53). Against the backdrop of severe illness and the fading of life outlined before, the outcome was very often an unfinished plot. Attempts at therapeutic emplotment which did not succeed, or succeeded only half way, will be the focus of the following considerations.

In the next story, I attempt to give coffee to Mrs Schauer, a patient with intestinal cancer in her fifties:

> She is lying in bed, in a very bad state. I ask about coffee and cake, a little coffee, she says, and that very moment I recall that she has severe problems with vomiting. Her husband, who is sitting beside her looking helpless suggests to ask the nurse. I pause to think and then turn to Mrs Schauer and tell her to decide by herself, whether it would be OK with the coffee or not, she could just taste a sip and then spit it out again. I pour a little into the feeding cup (which is always called a mug here), and then enter the room again [pouring being done at a trolley on the corridor]. The husband is still concerned, it's still too hot anyway, I say, wait five minutes, I will ask the nurse. Later I am told that she had to throw up after drinking the coffee.

Mrs Schauer liked the idea of having coffee. Once I realised there were possible obstacles, I tried to redirect her desire towards the experience of just tasting it – as in the previous story a pleasant experience was to be facilitated, and the practice of just tasting something was not unusual when patients could not eat or drink. The patient and I, against the cautioning of her husband, then started unravelling our projected plot of how she felt like drinking coffee; I gave her some in spite of her illness and she loved it. Unfortunately for us, instead she threw up and the whole attempt was thwarted: emplotment failed to produce positive experience.

In the first case of Mr Tanner, communication was possible, desire provoked, he started to participate in the developing plot suggested by staff, and the breakfast episode finishes with a feeling of success. The next example, Mrs Schauer's, finishes mid-way: she would like coffee, tries, but is unable to keep it. The story became a configured whole, an attempt was at least made, but it did not create positive experience.

In the following case of Mr Krieger, a patient with a brain tumour, not even such an initial development was possible:

> I take coffee and cake to Mr Krieger. He lies in bed motionless, one eye open, the other closed. If one is lucky, he opens both eyes when people are present. In case of pain or discomfort he makes a humming sound. I give him three biscuits for diabetics. This happens in the following manner, which in my eyes is typical for dealings with half-comatose people here. Hello Mr Krieger. No reaction. I have brought coffee and cake for you, would you like that? Slight, unspecific movement of the face. OK, I will put up the headrest of the bed [Ger.: Kopfteil] now, which I do. Mr Krieger still does not react, but now both his eyes are open. When the first biscuit touches his lips, he opens the mouth and slightly puts out the tongue, as old catholic peasant women do for the Holy Communion. Then he chews. I have the impression that it is all a little dry, and give him a sip of coffee with milk from the feeding cup. His open mouth at first does not change when the cup touches it, he hardly seems to notice the difference, after a while he sucks a little. This goes back and forth, I keep commenting and asking in between, does it taste OK, right, another biscuit, do you want more coffee, and he never reacts, just by opening the mouth and chewing. In the end I put the bed back into the lying position and say, well, that was it, see you later then. He lies there as before and I go away.

What can be observed are several attempts by me, the nurse, to draw him out and try to engage him to perceive coffee and biscuits as interesting. In order to engage him, I continuously addressed him, specifically by asking questions about whether he liked or wanted something, a question to which the answer could have been the starting point for an attempt to emplot the whole situation. I paid careful attention to his reactions and recorded them several times, trying to read non-verbal answers where verbal answers were not to be expected. However, from the patient's side, the only reactions remained chewing, swallowing and the opening of one eye.

There was no successful therapeutic emplotment in this case – all attempts got stuck at stage one. While there is my own story to tell, it never develops a shared plot. However, this makes the piece a particularly well suited example for nursing behaviour in that first stage, for the eliciting of desire and the attempt to guide that desire to some future goal. I have mentioned before that hospice nurses continuously addressed patients. Through this example, one goal of such behaviour becomes clear: continuous attempts to communicate ensure that the nurses can use every possible occasion to pick up the patient's desire and emplot the whole situation. At Mr Krieger's first reaction, I would probably have tried to get more biscuits, give him more coffee or follow up another desire that he might have voiced. Indeed, I would suggest that I told the story to my diary precisely because of the total absence of a reaction, which made the whole incident strange and thus worth relating.

My account of Mr Krieger is a striking example of what I have called the root consideration of the hospice movement in chapter one: to delay social death as much as possible and ideally not let it happen before biological death. I, the nurse, treat Mr Krieger as a full social person and do my best to elicit signs that he really is such a full person. Through my behaviour, I actively try to construct a communicative and practical situation in which it is possible not to consider him socially dead.

Just as conversation was geared to find possible starting points for therapeutic emplotment, food was prepared in a way that symbolised aesthetic enjoyment beyond just taste and nutrition:

> What impresses me is the affectionate presentation of the meals: Bernhard [kitchen staff] makes a great arrangement [Ger.: Arrangement], even for people with 'finely chopped food' who can hardly respond anymore [Ger.: ansprechbar sein]. An even, round scoop of mashed potatoes with a little valley in the middle for the sauce, three tiny pieces of liver draped onto this volcano, plus a little onion ring and two roast bits of apple. He does not seem to mind that only three bites of it will be eaten.

I was once told in a conversation by a nurse that the cook, when patients could not eat at all any more, would sometimes just cut pieces of vegetable into artistic forms to symbolise a meal that could at least be looked at with enjoyment.

Several stages were thus analysed in the discussion of therapeutic emplotment: the focus shifted from a complete, configured success story, to a story broken off in the middle, and then to a story that never started. Finally, on the most microscopic level, communication habits and symbols that could serve as starting points for stories were considered. In the experiential domain, a parallel movement can be seen from a positive breakfast experience, to an ambivalent attempt to drink coffee, on to a feeding interaction the experiential value of which for the patient remains unknown, and finally to words and symbols that are offered as possible catalysts for experience not yet present. In all these cases, I suggest that therapeutic emplotment was an important tool for nurses to counter those elements in fading life which threatened to lead to the social death of the patient. This will also become apparent in the following examples, which widen the scope again to longer sequences of interaction.

Mrs Hunn's Tour of the Hospice

A prominent goal of hospice nursing was the mobilisation of patients. When a patient first came to the hospice, nurses would always try to make her participate in meals in the communal kitchen. Getting there from patient's rooms often required some strength and either the straightforward admittance or the covering up of stigmatising outward signs of illness such as incontinence, visible growths and wounds, or erratic movement.

The patient about whom the next diary excerpt tells, a woman in her early eighties, refused to eat in the kitchen because her cancer of the oesophagus often made her throw up and she was ashamed of that. She had arrived in Stadtwald Hospice the day before and sat in a chair in her room without pursuing any apparent activity. Nurses were considering different methods to mobilise her and to get her out of her room.

> Today, I have little to do – nothing, in fact. While I sit there back in the staff room, Gerda comes along, has something to do there, and when she sees me she suggests, well, if you have nothing to do, why don't you go to Mrs Hunn and suggest to her going for a walk around the ward, only up to the newspapers [on a table in the middle section of the corridor], she is a very sociable person really, she just does not dare to go out [of her room], because she has to throw up so often. So a little while later I go to see Mrs Hunn. She must be in about her mid-eighties, has a cancer of the oesophagus, can only talk slowly, and, as has been said at handover, can hardly eat without having to vomit. I do not know her yet. When I come in she sits in the armchair; she has white hair and very dark brown eyes, at first I notice no signs of an illness. I am Nicholas, I say, nice to meet you, the nurse told me you might want to have a look at the ward? She seems quite happy about my offer. I notice by her hesitation that she is probably unable to stand up by herself. In front of her stands a walking frame. I approach her and support her under the arm, she tries to stand up but is too weak. She seems to lose confidence, I am too weak, she says with a low, coarse voice, the voice is affected by the cancer, I think. I stand directly in front of her, lean forward, put my arms around her and cross my hands behind her back. I am holding you completely safely now, we will stand up at three: one, two, three. Mrs Hunn can stand by herself all right. I ask whether it is OK for her to take the 'Rollator', or walk on my arm; she seems a little helpless and leans backward a bit, I support her quickly and she sits back into the chair again. Mrs Hunn, I ask, shall I get a wheelchair? Yes, she says, and seems relieved, yes.

The story starts not unlike the one about Mr Tanner's breakfast: a nurse suggested to me that I create an experience for a patient which was somewhat more than she would have expected. It could potentially increase her knowledge about her surroundings in the hospice and thus help her to locate herself in a life world. However, we encountered an obstacle: Mrs Hunn was weaker than I thought, maybe than she thought herself, which threatened the developing plot until I decided to change plans and get a wheelchair. This adaptation to changing circumstances is quite typical for nurses' dealing with fading life on patients' illness trajectories: the more experienced nurses often developed an almost detective-like ability to discover change and adapt to it quickly without giving off the impression that something negative, let alone something to be called a deterioration, had happened.

> So I go and get a wheelchair, transferring to the wheelchair works without problems, like standing up before. We set off. I ask Mrs Hunn, who has been here only for a couple of days, how often she has left her room, once, she says. I push her wheelchair very slowly and stop whenever there is something to see or to comment on, and I take care

to comment on anything that can be commented on at all. First we get to the kitchen, I say, well, that is the kitchen, have you seen it already, yes, says Mrs Hunn. Somebody greets us in passing, hello Mrs Hunn, nice to see you here, is this your first outing around the ward, the second, I say.

My continuous commenting can again be interpreted as an attempt to provide starting points for communication and material for the development of the therapeutic plot which has started to unravel. This in fact succeeded once we came to a window with a wide view over the city:

> We come to the roofed terrace, she finds that interesting, I follow a large, slow circle inside it. I was baptised in the church across there, she says while looking over the roofs. I am surprised, the church is only two blocks away, then you are from Altenberg here, I say, we continue to exchange a sentence or two, she talks in a very low voice and I have difficulties understanding, because I am standing behind the wheelchair, a real conversation does not start. She looks at everything with an expression of concentration. We pass the artificial decoration well with all the plants on the corridor, I tell her how once the sister of a patient who was here for very a long time put some fish inside, to feed them regularly. Yes, says Mrs Hunn, well, and I add that Liane, maybe you know her, added some more fish, who now live there. They are difficult to see, I say, they are behind the stone over there. Look, I change the position of the wheelchair, maybe you can see. Don't bother, says Mrs Hunn, I cannot see very well, I do not recognise anything. Ah, is that so, I say.

The view of the church opened up a possibility for conversation. With a stronger patient, it could have led to the suggestion to visit the church – a suggestion of a different, more ambitious turn in the therapeutic plot. However, that was impossible, and also my next move, an attempt to present the fishpond as very interesting, could not succeed against the backdrop of her failing eyesight.

> We go on, past the staff room, to the offices up front, I say a couple of sentences about everything, she notices the pictures on the walls, says a couple of words about them. We drive back along the corridor, I would like to read some names on the doors, says Mrs Hunn, I read one or two names to her: it almost seems as if she expected to know somebody. We pass Mrs Mertens's room, the door is wide open, we greet her warmly; Mrs Mertens just looks up briefly and says something like, I have things to do, which surprises me a bit in style and content. Shame, I would have liked for the two of them to get to know each other, I hope Mrs Hunn does not regret it as much as I do.

Mrs Hunn's interest in learning about the names of the occupants of other rooms demonstrates some interest in her social surroundings, but my hope to give the plot a new turn by introducing her to Mrs Mertens failed.

> When we come back to her room she seems to expect to go in again, because she looks that way instead of down the corridor, we can, if you want, go down to the other end

of the corridor, I say, no problem. OK, we go on to the living room, where I say something about the smokers who use it, and then back to her room. I help her into her armchair, ask whether she has any wishes, no, says Mrs Hunn, it was very nice, thanks a lot. She seems happy and tired. Well, until later then, I say goodbye and go.

Once the action got started, I myself as the nurse tried my best to prolong it, to provide some extra plot and further occasions for communication and interaction. In this context it is interesting how many of the judgements I made about whether Mrs Hunn is satisfied or not seem to be based at least as much on my hopes and desires, namely to construct a meaningful experience for her, than on her own. She remained the passive partner in the account and I succeeded only very occasionally in involving her in the plot. This tendency continued during the following days, where I displayed an activating attitude, trying to mobilise her and to get her involved:

> Somebody says in the staff room, Mrs Hunn did not have to throw up at all today, you know, great, I say, then maybe she can go to the kitchen to eat from now on, no, says the other person, she is too afraid she might still have to throw up then.

On one of the following days, I attempted to start another story by suggesting that she sit in the sun on the terrace. However, this was countered by the progression of her disease.

> Today, the sun really shines for the first time this spring. I distribute coffee and cake with Leo. When I am in Mrs Hunn's room, it occurs to me that I could sit her out on the terrace. So I ask, Mrs Hunn, would it be an idea to sit in the sun on the terrace, I could help you in a short while, with the wheelchair or whatever, how would you like that? Yes, says Mrs Hunn, and looks happy. OK, I say, then I will come back later and we will do that.
>
> After we have finished [distributing] coffee I ask Gerda what she thinks of my idea, yes, she says, good, why don't you do that. A little later the bell rings, number nine [room numbers appear on a display outside the staff room], Mrs Hunn, great coincidence. I go to her room and say something energetic like, OK Mrs Hunn, let's start, yes, she says, I am very tired and I have to go to bed. The plan with the terrace does not materialise: I help her to bed.

Mrs Hunn was quite a typical example of how bodily and mental changes fused in one process of her whole person fading away. When she arrived at the hospice, there were no outward signs of the illness, she could walk short distances and seemed aware, if a bit slow in her communication. There still seemed to be a possibility to counteract the process through offering communication, interaction and mobility, as possible starting point of a shared, emplotted experience. However, already at this point Mrs Hunn remained quite passive, too weak to pick up the suggestions and soon too weak for sensible suggestions to be made. During the week or two of her stay, she rapidly lost both strength and interest in her surroundings, was soon confined to bed, stopped speaking, became incontinent, and died.[6]

Grand Schemes – A Nurses' Dispute

Emplotment, always being implicit anyway, was not a uniform, rigid strategy in a fixed hospice nursing repertoire, but rather an attitude and practice about which there could be as much agreement or disagreement between staff as about any other aspect of nursing. In fact, novice nurses such as myself tended to attempt much grander emplotment schemes aiming at much more spectacular success stories than experienced nurses, who would ground their attempts in the more mundane details of everyday life. While the more experienced were often content when they succeeded in constructing eating or washing as meaningful experiences, novices taken in by the hospice ways sometimes attempted to facilitate much more ambitious projects. The following episode is about a conflict between a novice nurse and two more experienced staff.

Mr Lehmann was a man in his sixties who had cancer of the kidneys and suffered from the beginning neurological consequences of a drinking habit. He was still able to look after himself alone and while he got weaker, he could walk short distances without support or supervision. His partner had a physical disability which apparently did not allow her to visit him in the hospice.

> During the course of the week Thomas has mentioned that tomorrow he would drive Mr Lehmann to see his partner, at eleven, because she could not come to visit Mr Lehmann herself due to some sort of disability. All this has supposedly been checked with the manager. When, at handover, we get to Mr Lehmann, [room] number four, Anne [nurse on nightshift] recounts what happened during the night, how it was known that Mr Lehmann appeared to be much weaker this week, and how the outing was planned for today. Micha, who was on the nightshift with Anne, quite suddenly addresses Thomas and asks: does Mr Lehmann really want all that? What do you mean, does he want that, Thomas replies, well, does he want it himself, is he fit for it? A long discussion follows, in which Anne and Micha on the one hand question whether Mr Lehmann has the strength to go [up the stairs] to an apartment on the fourth floor, and Thomas on the other hand finds himself pushed into the defence with his attempt to reunite Mr Lehmann and his partner for one last time. Edeltraud tries to mediate, Gert, Erika, Rita and myself say nothing, but, as we discuss later, all find the style of Anne and Micha a little unfair. For me, the whole discussion sounds as if Thomas was being charged with having initiated the whole outing, for which Mr Lehmann was too weak, all by himself. Several scenarios are discussed, taxi or medical transportation service [Ger.: Krankentransport], or maybe a third person to come along; many objections are voiced, but Thomas insists on his project – if Mr Lehmann wants that, he will do it, if not, he will cancel it, where is the problem? However, he

never says clearly what kind of wish it was that Mr Lehman had told him about. Later during the day it turns out, Mr Lehmann does not want to go after all, and Thomas says, well, that's OK, for Mr Lehmann it was all about thinking it over, really.

The story started at handover. Thomas, the novice nurse, failed to enlist support amongst his colleagues for a rather ambitious meaning-making project, namely to bring together Mr Lehmann and his partner for one last time outside of the hospice. He had apparently prepared this for quite some time. Two experienced nurses, Anne and Micha, questioned the whole idea and claimed that the patient was too weak to undertake such a visit. Several scenarios were drawn up and discussed. Typically, the discussion did not become categorical and resort to authority. Neither did Anne and Micha refer directly to their own status as far more experienced, better trained and higher up in the hierarchy, which they were, nor did they call on the manager or the senior nurse to resolve the conflict. In the end, it was left to the patient himself finally to reject the idea.

At the time of writing my diaries, I took it for granted that the patient had indeed voiced the clear wish to see his partner at her home, and I rejected Anne and Micha's suggestion that it might all have been Thomas's idea in the first place. Thomas himself in the end claimed that 'for Mr Lehmann, thinking about it was the important thing, really'. With the hindsight of the emplotment perspective, I would now interpret the occasion differently and consider my own position at the time a bit naive. Probably Mr Lehmann had indeed said something about wanting to see his partner, but given his weakness and occasional confusion it seems unlikely to me that he drew up the whole scenario of the visit all by himself. Rather, it could have been Thomas who tried to emplot an initial desire into the grand narrative of the last rendezvous he facilitated for the dying patient, involving Mr Lehmann in it with gentle and indirect persuasion. In this scenario, Anne and Micha, who had more experience about what kind of meaning-making projects were still feasible for Mr Lehmann, rightly became suspicious that the whole project was maybe more about Thomas's needs than about those of the patient. In all this, I do not think that Thomas was aware of what he was trying to do and why; he was probably genuinely convinced that it all was Mr Lehmann's idea and only in his best interests.

If emplotment in the hospice context was about drawing patients out of the general fading away of their life for a little while, this story also illustrates that it took quite a bit of experience and measure to judge patients' situations correctly, design the right plot and carry it through. When a nurse's own desire to help combined with a lack of experience, there could be a risk that an emplotment attempt would become overbearing for the patient. However, that tended to be the exception during my fieldwork periods, and most nurses had a very accurate feeling, developed through years of experience, of what was still possible to do and what was not.

Challenges for Mr Kasparek

Already in the discussion of the accounts of Mr Tanner's breakfast and Mrs Hunn's tour of the hospice, the headings of 'food' and 'mobility' under which the stories were presented only highlight a central, but by no means the only, activity present. Mr Tanner did not just eat, he also smoked, talked, and through conversation considered the impending visit of his wife. In a similar vein, Mrs Hunn did not just relocate from A to B, but, in a limited way, engaged in conversation, revisited childhood memories, and was made aware of the social setting she found herself in. In both cases, therapeutic emplotment started out from a nursing task such as providing food, or pushing a wheelchair. Through the creation of desire the plot then gradually grew to involve many aspects of both patients' life worlds. Emplotment tried to reconstruct such life worlds against the backdrop of their fading.

Just as fading life encompassed the whole person, the emplotment attitude tried temporarily to reconstruct the life world through reaching out for the whole person, assuming that physical improvement would lead to mental well-being and vice versa. In the discussion of the following, longer accounts of Mr Kasparek, I will not so much look at emplotment in the narrower sense analysed above. Rather, informed by the emplotment perspective, I shall presently widen the view to a more general analysis of how nurses tried to counter fading life by reconstructing a life world for a patient.

Mr Kasparek is about forty years old, it was said, likes football and weight training, and is paralysed from the waist downwards, probably a consequence of radiotherapy because of his lung cancer. He has strong inner tensions and trembles a lot. Yesterday he apparently almost collapsed while being wheeled back from the shower into his room in a shower chair [Ger.: Duschstuhl].

We go into the room, chat a little. Mr Kasparek is visibly nervous, we help him to undress, there is a little blood in his incontinence pad, it is not quite clear why. Mr Kasparek has a very muscular build and is quite strong, one or two tattoos, not very professionally done. He tries hard to help us but that does not always work, the paralysis starts quite high up at the waist. Together, we lift him into a chair, Dieter with Rautek-Griff [a specific type of grasp for lifting], while I take the legs, all works well. Mr Kasparek then says, the occasional smell of urine drives me mad, we are used to it and tell him that, Dieter wants to avoid that the hardly noticeable smell should embarrass him, I think. Then Dieter leaves, as Mrs Ohlsen must be looked after, and I shower Mr Kasparek. That goes quite well: he relaxes visibly, we take our time and chat a little in between. It becomes clear how very much his situation, being dependent, frustrates him. Probably, I think, he was always a very strong and independent, traditional type of man.

After quite some time I push his wheelchair back into the room, Dieter comes to help, and it is back into bed. Then Liane, whom we call, renews the bandage for the bedsores. Dieter then talks with Mr Kasparek about his situation, he explains to him in a direct yet understanding manner how he should now concentrate on his legs, that's training, you are a sportsman, you know how it is: even with hard work you don't get immediate results, but still you have to train. Mr Kasparek listens to that and does seem somewhat grateful, saying in between yes, that's the way it is, it does not come easy, but he would try, better than staring at the ceiling, you know. When we leave, he is in a much better mood, very tired as well. That shower was really nice, he says.

In the account, Mr Kasparek enjoyed having a shower. Helping him to have showers in order to facilitate enjoyment subsequently became a key event in his care. There is also, in the diary excerpt, an example of how he was encouraged by the nurse to become more active and self-reliant: he had worked hard on his physical fitness before his illness, and nurse Dieter tried an appeal to his sportsman's ethos, telling him to train and see whether he could regain command of his legs. The aim of this intervention was probably to give him a general feeling that he could improve his situation through a combination of effort and acceptance – a theme of hospice nursing discussed previously. At the time, I was rather taken aback by what I considered quite a demanding thing to ask of a paralysed patient.

However, similar to Dieter, another much more experienced nurse named Walter saw activation and especially mobilisation as crucial goals in the overall treatment of Mr Kasparek. The following diary excerpt has been discussed previously as an example of images of the hospital, but is considered in its larger context here:

Afterwards on the corridor I ask Walter what the point of a suprapubic catheter is, he says it is less infectious than one via the urethra. He explains some other things in Mr Kasparek's clinical picture [Ger.: Krankheitsbild], and while he stays outwardly calm he does get a bit worked up about it. He says he is angry because, in the hospital, quite a number of things had been done wrong with Mr Kasparek. First, the patient contracted a bladder infection, which could be detected by the particles in his urine, and something like that was completely superfluous. The way he phrases it, it sounds as if the hospital had actually made the bladder infection. Then, he had never been mobilised, which gave him bedsores [on the lower back], and intestinal problems, because he had not been allowed to sit on the toilet, but been given strong laxatives and a napkin instead. This in turn led to semi-liquid excrements [Ger.: schmieriger Stuhl], which of course was no good for the bedsores. Besides all this there were the psychological problems, which a situation like that caused for a man like him. It was now of crucial importance to mobilise him as often as possible, in order to make the bedsores go away and get to grips with the intestinal problem in a less aggressive fashion.

In the text, lack of activity and attention are presented by the nurse as the trigger for a causal chain reaching from a bladder infection to severe psychological problems. The start of it all is blamed on the hospital. Mobilisation is presented as the key remedy and, in the following days, it ranked high on the nurses' agenda. They did succeed at first:

> Dieter is determined today to mobilise Mr Kasparek: yesterday this was prevented by his weakness, he would really like it in fact. Later, when I come to the kitchen to help distribute lunch, Mr Kasparek is sitting there, at the table with Mrs Sartorius, Mrs Marx and Gertrud [cleaning staff]. They are having a lively conversation and seem in a good mood, I join them for a while and have lunch myself: Königsberger Klopse [traditional German meatball dish] with potatoes. Very nice, especially the potatoes, says Mrs Sartorius. Then I sit in the staff room, the door bell rings, it is Mr Kasparek's brother, who I go to receive at the lift, so that he does not get frightened when he finds the room is empty; I tell him that Mr Kasparek is in the kitchen. The two of them then go and sit in the room. Shortly before handover, Dieter and I go there again, to offer to lift Mr Kasparek into bed, but with Dieter adding that he does not think that would make too much sense. Mr Kasparek agrees wholeheartedly, he wants to remain seated, we leave again. On the corridor Dieter laughs and says, that's a success isn't it, the way the man felt this morning and his good mood now. We both agree that the trembling is probably psychological [Ger.: psychisch]; I propose it also might have to do with his former training, muscle tension and all that, but that's not the main issue here.

On the day of the excerpt presented, nurses succeeded for the first time during his stay at Stadtwald Hospice to mobilise Mr Kasparek. Subsequently, he spent the day in a wheelchair, had lunch in the communal kitchen, met some other patients, talked to his brother, and had not gone back to bed by the time the shift ended, preferring to remain seated in the wheelchair. We, the nurses, were delighted about all this, thinking probably correctly that we had succeeded in significantly enriching the experience of a patient formerly confined to a hospital bed. From then on, Mr Kasparek continued to eat in the communal kitchen and meet patients and staff there.

> Mr Kasparek has an active day today, he is in the kitchen for lunch, and tries to joke with Mrs Sartorius, which does not go so well: he seems a little too deliberate to me. After the meal, for a smoke, we bring him to the living room, where a couple of nurses sit and smoke, he joins. I fetch his cigarettes from his room, he offers them to everybody even though they all have their own, and then he stays for a while.

My overall summary that he 'had an active day' is typical hospice nursing jargon. An active day was what patients were encouraged to have, after all. A certain ambivalence remained, however, about the social interaction he engaged in, as his efforts were received with some distance by staff and the unusually independent Mrs Sartorius. The last statement I found in my diaries sums up quite neatly how, from the hospice perspective, nurses' work with Mr Kasparek had been successful:

Today I look after Mr Kasparek again: a shower, taking showers is important to him and he enjoys it a lot, we take him for a shower almost every day. Afterwards, he is always quite relaxed, perhaps for the only time in the day. Once he complains his sister was so dominant and always talked so much. We talk about this for a while, the sister really seems to get on his nerves, she is bossy, he says.

We find that over a period of maybe a week or so, nurses had succeeded in forging a shared success story in which Mr Kasparek came to go along with central values of hospice nursing: at first, nurses found out that he enjoyed showers and immediately made that pleasant experience a central point of his care. Then, he was mobilised and enabled to interact socially. Finally, he came to confide in the nurses about personal problems and thus entered into a relationship of one-sided emotional disclosure which was very typical for the hospice context.

In all of these areas, some reservations remained: concerning the showers, they sometimes made Mr Kasparek too weak and sleepy to remain active. Also, he still was quite awkward in social interaction. Finally, the problem about his relationship with his sister was often discussed with the nurses, but could not be rectified, for he never found the courage to approach the topic directly with her.

As my fieldwork period ended at that time, I have little further information about Mr Kasparek. He died in the hospice some weeks afterwards. At the point where my account of him breaks off, it is a success story from the hospice point of view. Against the backdrop of fading life, nurses succeeded to draw him out of the isolated situation in his room, make him interact with others and have pleasant experiences. A different life world was temporarily reconstructed by the way he and the nurses interacted and fused their goals and desires into one common project. Single initiatives within that project were guided by the emplotment attitude, while the overall result was eminently practical and concrete.

It remains open for interpretation whether therapeutic emplotment in a narrower sense was relevant in this broader account over time, but the attitude displayed by nurses throughout this example, the goals and underlying values of their actions, bear a lot of resemblance to the more text-based analysis of emplotment in the earlier sections of this chapter. Most importantly, however, the account of Mr Kasparek shows that an emplotment attitude could have results that were very concrete and well beyond an understanding of narratives as simply textual representation removed from actual social life.

No Stories to Tell – Failure Revisited

I have already discussed the observation that nurses would not be able to tell me about a time when they perceived their work as failed. It was suggested that, in addition to very flexible, patient-centred attitudes, the fading of life ultimately forced patients to give in to the nurses' will anyway. However, this turns out to be only one possible perspective. From the point of view of narrative anthropology and therapeutic emplotment, another perspective can now be taken on failure and its peculiar absence at Stadtwald Hospice.

As has been demonstrated, success was seen in the interactive construction of meaningful or pleasant experiences, based on a reflexive, aware and active self, using narrative structures. A story to tell was a success. Even when such stories failed, that was always due to the inevitable general fading of life. Thus, an emplotment attempt which failed half-way was at least a good try and in the patients' best interests, anyway. What about the times when there was no story, though?

In my diaries, from which I have so far mostly quoted configured stories, there are also a number of small fragments, hardly emplotted enough to call them narratives, which hint at all those patients who never made it into my field notes because there was no story to tell about them. These fragments appear not for their own sake, but because they provide some background for other events I described. One of them features Mr Meise, who also appears at the sidelines of some other stories:

> A certain Mr Meise has been admitted recently, it seems as if he were connected to a lot of technical equipment, but he is apparently conscious and clearly aware of his situation [Ger.: orientiert]. It must have been a lot of work to prepare all that equipment, and he cannot talk. I get the impression Mr Meise is a difficult case.
>
> ...
>
> Renate [the hospice manager] is there today, partly sits in at handover, then discusses problems with the staff rota with Kerstin. I approach her briefly, about how to proceed in March, she says that of course the more I worked the better it would be for her, 'because that way we get to know you well' [Ger.: vertraut werden] Apart from that there is not much to say. When we talk about medicine as part of my work she mentions a couple of pointless machines, including an internal body thermometer, which they had removed from Mr Meise on his arrival here.
>
> ...
>
> In any case, suddenly there is some dramatic incident, as I am told later, with Mr Meise – I do not understand of which kind – and Greta and the doctor are completely busy with that and pass the rest of the work on to Kerstin and myself.
>
> ...
>
> Mr Meise has died and is already gone. He was here for just two days.

Mr Meise is never mentioned for his own sake. The first narrative is really about handover. The second one is about a conversation with the hospice manager and about biomedical equipment. The third one serves as explanation why I had an unusual amount of work one day. In the fourth bit, which is from a standard account of a handover, Mr Meise has already died. Considering hospice statistics, there must have been many patients like him, hardly mentioned in my diaries.

The presence of patients like Mr Meise gives an additional explanation for the absence of accounts of failure: While success – experience, interaction, enjoyment – was narratively structured, failure simply did not lend itself to narrativisation and emplotment. It remained an absence in any account. When there was no discernible desire or motivation, no human agency and no plot, no obstacles to overcome and no goals to reach, and no change from chronological to emplotted time, then hospice aspirations maybe could be said to have failed. In such cases, however, there was no narrative to tell, and simply no story to remember.

This consideration also shows the limits of narrative anthropology as a methodological and theoretical framework. In hindsight, it appears to me that there were many times when hospice nurses, including myself, would pass over odd, apparently unexplainable behaviour with a shrug, or interact with inaccessible patients from a benevolent distance. Depending on individual preferences, they would then largely refrain from activation, emplotment, and interaction. However, few stories remained to tell about such incidents.

This can be illustrated further with the example of Mr Blaschke, one patient who also appears as background to a story I wrote down about two nurses:

> Mr Blaschke is a patient of around seventy years, who can do almost everything [in daily life] by himself and does nothing without being told to. Sometimes he reasons clearly, other times again he talks total nonsense, but that hardly confuses me any more. Jojo knows, and tells me to go and have a look every now and then, to see if Mr Blaschke eats, and to tell him to get dressed, or to undress. When he lies in bed, Mr Blaschke wraps himself into a bare woollen blanket without touching the normal duvet, I point it out to him – sometimes people forget these things – but he just says, it's all right this way. I feel a strange kind of distant appreciation, but at the same time I somehow do not really care. Later on in the corridor, Steffen and Jojo joke about the typical hand gesture of the hospice nurse; Steffen makes a mocking, resigned gesture with his hand, as if throwing something over his shoulder, they laugh.

Mr Blaschke, in all he does, casually refuses to engage in the creation of shared experience. Typically, this is the only time his name appears in my diaries, while there are many pages about other patients who did occasion shared experiences. The nurses tolerated Mr Blaschke with sympathy; he was not asked to do anything, but looked at with a sort of benevolent, resigned distance.

The two nurses mentioned in the diary excerpt see this benevolent distance as a typical attitude of hospice nursing. This attitude was, in fact, the other, hidden side of the emplotment coin, and it was relatively widespread. It had a lot to do with the unpredictable circumstances of fading life, which often forced nurses to adopt an accepting, 'phenomenological' approach to patients' behaviours rather than an analytical, prescriptive one. Being able to suspend assumptions could make it easier for them to work and led to an acceptance of those patients who were simply there, occasioning no special experiences for anybody and no narratives to tell.

Notes

1. In a slightly different context Walter (1994: 69) points out that stories are the main format of revivalist talk, that is, of the discourse of those who propagate a 'new' interest in death.

2. In what follows, I present my own brief synthesis of the ideas of the three authors mentioned above. These authors in turn owe some debt to the narrative current in social psychology as represented by Jerome Bruner, in Mattingly's case also to the hermeneutic tradition of Paul Ricoeur (1981) and to the 'Harvard School' of medical anthropology (e.g. Kleinman 1988, Good 1994). Arnason (1998: 33–37) and especially Mattingly (1998: 6–47) provide a good summary presentation of the narrative approach. Mattingly also discusses in great detail what positions are at stake in epistemology, hermeneutics and literary theory. With respect to narrative in ethnography, see also Sal Buckler's recent study on gypsies in north east England (in press).

3. See chapter one for details about Kübler-Ross. Sogyal Rimpoche is a Tibetan Buddhist teacher with a very wide following in the West who has written extensively on death and dying in the context of the Tibetan Book of The Dead, a traditional text. See Sogyal (2004) for one edition amongst many.

4. Fernandez (1986: 15) makes an analogous observation about the use of figurative speech in conflict resolution amongst the Fang, a non-hierarchical African people: in a largely egalitarian society where there is no effective hierarchy to enforce judgments, he argues, careful ambiguity of statement is required. Aphorisms, proverbs and metaphors provide ways of commenting upon the essentials of experience in one domain by extending these essentials to analogous experiences in another domain. The essential wisdom of the comment may be preserved in the extension while a painful and possibly unenforceable precision is obscured.

5. Neither do I say that the bottle he was finally content with was one anatomically suited for women. I found that out when going over this incident with nurses later in the staff room, to their great amusement.

6. I have commented elsewhere (Eschenbruch 2005) on the relevance of material objects for my tour with Mrs Hunn, an aspect that is not so central here.

5
DEATH AT
STADTWALD HOSPICE

In the best case, what could be achieved through approaches such as therapeutic emplotment in a hospice situation was to make social and biological death coincide as much as possible and to make the remaining time worth living for the patient. However, both approximations of death remained ultimately inevitable. The last ethnographic chapter of this study is thus concerned with the immediate social surroundings of death and cultural arrangements concerning it at Stadtwald Hospice.[1] The framework of narrative ethnography and the understanding of my material as stories will of course remain, but rather than applying one particular theory, I will make reference to theoretical points already made and to results already obtained in the previous chapters.[2]

Arrangements Surrounding Death

If individual patients' trajectories at the hospice are seen as stories, as mutually co-constructed, emplotted configurations, then experienced nurses knew about the final outcome of such stories well in advance. From their point of view, patients' stories converged more and more towards the end; individual differences became less as life faded. In the emplotment perspective it could be said that, while the exact course of the unravelling plot was unpredictable and at times contested, nurses knew much better than patients what the end of the story would be like. As one nurse remarked to me retrospectively about a patient who had refused completely to wash, shave or undertake any measures of personal hygiene: 'Towards the end, it became easier to look after him'.

Nurses also had clear ideas as to when the last phase of the narrative started. There were a number of signs that showed to nurses that a patient did not have much longer to live: one nurse told me that 'confusion and restlessness plus two days' was her rule of thumb as to how long someone would still live. She explained that this had to do, biomedically speaking, with multiple organ failure and an accumulation of toxic substances in the body. A pale, 'sharp' nose and the formation of a pale, triangular area on an unconscious patient's face was seen as an even closer indicator, pointing to a death likely to occur soon, probably within the next couple of hours. Finally, deep gasping breaths with long interruptions in between served as a similar sign. When nurses interpreted such signs, their biomedical knowledge about them combined with their experience of having seen them in many patients – and also came with a clear awareness that all these signs could be misleading.

The connotation of 'dying' in the internal hospice usage was quite different from the social construction of a life phase 'dying' as discussed in the first chapter: for hospice staff, patients were 'dying' when their death was imminent, likely to occur within hours, maybe within two or three shifts at the most. There is a certain discrepancy here between the general assumption of the hospice movement – a long dying phase calls for special institutions – and the inside understanding that dying was a short matter, and the preceding phase just a phase of life. In actual practice, signs of approaching death did not necessarily alter nursing routines and were often taken with a caring, but quite matter-of-fact attitude. This is shown by the following text, which was written one day before the patient who is described in it died:

> Around noon, before handover, I am in Mr Haller's room with Kerstin, to wash him and change the bandages for his renal catheters. I realise that I have learned to identify a Tjelle® [a specific brand of adhesive bandage for bedsores], Mr Haller has one on his bedsore. He is not well, his breathing bubbles [sign of fluids in the bronchial tubes; Ger.: brodelt] and he does not react to us any more [Ger.: ist nicht ansprechbar]. At one point during washing his breathing changes suddenly, becomes much softer and less bubbly, I notice immediately and it reminds me of Mrs Rösch [a patient who had just died]; Kerstin says very calmly and in a quietly compassionate way, well, he won't leave us, will he, but continues her work just the same.

Whether a dying patient needed special attention was decided depending on their individual circumstances. The staff rota of a particular shift had to be taken into consideration, and generally nurses would see to it that patients were not alone in the last hours of their life. When somebody was both still conscious and very afraid, staff would be with them almost without interruption, even when that caused a considerable increase in work load for the other members of the nursing team. When death was approaching very slowly, however, as was often the case in unconscious brain tumour patients, nurses just checked on the patient regularly and tried to spend more time just being in the room.

If possible, the person staying with the patient would be a hospice staff member who had a closer relationship with that particular patient. This could be a nurse, but also administrative staff or volunteers, or, as in the diary excerpt below, cleaning staff. In fact, the full-time cleaner had an important and openly acknowledged role at Stadtwald Hospice in caring for patients who preferred a direct and hands-on attitude to the careful and considerate approach of many nurses. The following account is quite typical for what happened at the deathbed of hospice patients:

> Julia sends me to Mrs Struck, where I sit for an hour, because she is very poorly. When I enter, I am at first a little frightened: the grey-brownish colour of her face has made me nervous before, now her eyes are half closed and rolled away; she breathes in gasps, sometimes bubbly [Ger.: brodelnd], and does not react any more [Ger.: ist nicht mehr ansprechbar]. For a moment I consider saying that I do not want to sit with her, but then I stay; the fear dissolves and is replaced by compassion, but not warmth. In between Anne comes in and brings stuff for mouth care, Mrs Struck's lips are all chapped. Anne puts Bepanthen® ointment on them and we remove some bits of skin tissue. I keep sitting there, sometimes put my hand on the duvet and very softly move it onto hers, which is lying on her stomach. Her nose seems very white, the breathing a little weaker. Later, Monika [a cleaner] comes in and asks whether she could stay maybe, in fact I do not mind, but she seems insecure. I ask whether she has time, and she says, I would leave behind three rooms [that need cleaning] for that. She says she really liked Mrs Struck and asks me again whether she could stay, of course I say, no problem, and leave. When I pass by next time, there is a 'do not disturb' sign on the door.

First of all, once nurses decided that death was imminent, an auxiliary member of staff – myself – whose absence was felt less in the shift was sent into the room to be with the dying patient. At this point, nursing care had already been reduced to a minimum, sometimes even the strain of washing or changing incontinence pads could have led to the death of a patient. This minimum amount of nursing included all those tasks which made the situation a little more comfortable for patients. In the above case, a nurse put moisturising ointment on the patient's mouth, which typically became very dry at that point. Some form of physical contact with the patient was usually part of sitting by their deathbed. Some nurses claimed they could sense whether this was welcome or unwelcome to unconscious patients. Finally, it was quite typical that the person present during the last hours would be somebody who wanted this and felt close to the patient, in this case Monika, a member of the cleaning staff. My personal emotional reaction to this particular patient, a slight feeling of anxiety and an ambivalence as to whether I was supposed to be there, of course depended on the patient concerned. Mrs Struck died within a few hours after the events described, in the presence of Monika.

Relatives showed a wide range of reactions to impending death, as would be expected. Some wanted to be called any time and came rushing to the hospice when they were informed that matters were getting worse; others explicitly stated that they did not want to be present. There was a remark in every patient's file as to whether or not relatives wanted to be called when death seemed imminent. In such cases, nurses would make every effort to call them. However, since signs of approaching death were never unambiguous and relatives sometimes difficult to reach, their presence was not always possible.

Before relatives' last meeting with a patient, during her death and afterwards, nurses would try to support relatives as much as possible, by talking to them or by just being present and available. The following narrative tells about a death which, from the hospice perspective, went well:

> Mr Lerner gets worse around noontime, which is noticeable by his breathing – it now goes in gasps, starts to bubble and seems forced, but stays regular. A nurse calls Mrs Lerner, who arrives soon after. A little later I meet Mrs Lerner on the corridor; she says the breathing has changed again, is weaker now, I should have a look. I say someone who knows should do that, and I get Hartmut, they both go into the room. A few minutes later I hear that Mr Lerner has died in the presence of his wife and Hartmut. Mrs Lerner passes by the staff room a little later, she has to go and see the undertaker; she says she will show her appreciation later, we say she should not worry about that: there were more important things for her right now. She seems even paler than usual, but composed, a relative is with her.

I refer Mrs Lerner to a more senior nurse in such an important matter – a point stated in chapter two as characterising my research position in fieldwork. It is no coincidence that the account shifts to the relatives once death has been described. Since they had to start organising the funeral almost immediately, the time at the hospice directly after death was the only time some relatives would have at all between the long and tiring strain of severe illness and the social and administrative demands of death arrangements. Often, experienced nurses would talk things over with them at this point and offer emotional support.

Once the relatives had gone – or before they came if they arrived after death – the nurses would prepare the body of the dead person. One patient had died from a brain tumour only minutes after nurses and relatives had last seen him – below is the account of how we prepared his body afterwards:

> Mr Beaujean is to be prepared, and after a short consideration about who should do it I join Kerstin and Alexandra. We take a candle lamp with us and a small flower arrangement, which we put in front of the door. Then we enter the room. First, Kerstin and Alexandra remove the catheter, then Mr Beaujean gets a fresh incontinence pad. Then we dress him in normal clothes [he had been wearing a patients' gown which made nursing procedures easier]. The dead Mr Beaujean seems very peaceful to me, the weight of the illness seems to have fallen off. Alexandra suggests that I wear

gloves if all this disturbed me, not at all, I say, which is correct: the idea seems rather superstitious to me, as if corpses were infectious by their nature. The atmosphere is quiet, but not heavy, there is even a short playful remark or two. Mr Beaujean is still warm; we lift him up and turn him a little, to be able to put his clothes on him. All bedcovers are changed, a fresh pillow is prepared and a bedcover put over him [up to the shoulders]. Then a flower is put in his hand, from a visitors' bouquet which is in the room, the two nurses prefer that to a hospice flower, which Alexandra had already brought. A Buddha postcard, which was also on the desk, is put on the pillow next to him, and the picture of a boy, underneath which is written, 'Pierre, you know I will always be with you'. Alexandra says 'whatever that is' about the Buddha postcard, which means she does not recognise the religious connotation. Finally all the visible medical and nursing equipment is taken away, and then we leave. The window is open, there is a little wind and the curtains billow softly, but far into the room, which Alexandra and I notice, and we look at each other. Look, the curtains, she says, yes, I saw that too. Then we go to call the doctor and the relatives.

As shown in the above account, it was customary for deceased patients to have their hands folded over their chest, flowers were usually put somewhere on the bed, and articles of personal significance put on the night table next to it. The eyes of dead patients were closed when necessary, but the mouth and jaw were not bound up. All medical equipment was removed from the patient's body and from the room. The fact that the body of a patient was prepared in such way at all suggests that social relations with that person were not finished yet, a point to which I shall return later.

In this account, a couple of further points deserve attention: the first is the offer by nurse Alexandra that I put on rubber gloves when handling the corpse, which I considered unusual at the time. Both nurses were not wearing gloves, but apparently one of them assumed that relative newcomers would find touching a corpse problematic. I initially thought this was an idiosyncrasy of this nurse, but Pfeffer (1998: 126–33), in her detailed discussion of standard hospital practices, points out that it is the customary thing to do in hospital nursing when handling corpses.

A second interesting point is that the nurse did not recognise the Buddhist picture as a religious item, again suggesting that the formal symbolic language of religion was not prominent in Stadtwald Hospice. Finally, there is a moment at the end of the account when apparently both the nurse and myself considered the sudden movement of the curtains symbolic in some vaguely mystical way. However, it is again significant for the hospice approach that we neither denied the relevance of such symbolism, nor found it necessary to do anything about it beyond the pointing out.

Customarily, a candle was then put in front of the door, together with some flowers. While a dead person was in the hospice, a candle was also lit in a designated, centrally located corner opposite the staff room. Staff and visitors mostly saw the candles as a positive, dignified and indeed practical symbol – after all, it was quite functional to announce the presence of a dead person, so that relatives or staff would not rush into a room and be surprised. Patients, however, did not always appreciate the open acknowledgement of death through the candles, and a few of them really disliked the implicit reminder of their own situation:

> Mrs Marx, I learn, has a phobia concerning candles, because she knows what a candle in front of a room means: that a dead person is in there. She gets very tense and sad when she sees candles, the nurses tell me, and can only stand any other candles, even those for decoration, with great difficulty. When the storyteller comes, for example, and candles are put in the living room for atmosphere, Mrs Marx does not enjoy the tales at all and just gets irritated about the candles. She appreciates it when it is made possible for her not to be on the corridor as long as candles are there, and especially when the undertakers are about.

As has been mentioned in the discussion of informed consent in chapter two, it was never quite clear how aware patients were of their own situation, and, if they were, whether they wanted to be reminded of it at all. Similarly, the symbolism and ritual with which hospice staff surrounded death was not always welcomed by all patients. While death was by no means concealed at the hospice, and some staff made a point of making it visible, some patients themselves chose not to deal with the issue openly.

Farewells and Farewell Rituals

There was a wide consensus at the hospice that one ought to 'say farewell' [Ger.: sich verabschieden] to a dead patient if any kind of closer relationship had been established. However, the form of this farewell depended a lot on the nature and intensity of the relationship. When a patient had only been at the hospice for a day or two when she died, some nurses would maybe go into the room individually and chose their own form of farewell. In the case of patients who had been in the hospice for longer, more elaborate and communal forms were employed. Those were usually referred to as a 'Farewell' or, more often, 'the Ritual' [Ger.: Verabschiedung, das Ritual].[3]

Normally, it was asked at handover who of the nurses wanted to do the preparations for the Ritual and who wanted to participate. Generally speaking, it was customary to attend for those nurses who felt they had had a significant relationship with the patient in question. Administrative staff were often asked to participate as well.

The first Ritual I attended went as follows:

> Mrs Spitze has been prepared in the same way as Mr Bullinger: hands on the stomach, but not folded, a flower between them. Her chin has not been bound up, when I ask, Tanja says that everything was meant to be 'really natural'; later I learn that the rigor

mortis partly closes the mouth again anyway. First the brother and his wife enter the room, then we do. We position ourselves spread out around the room. Then Tanja steps forward a little and says 'Today, we want to say farewell to Mrs Spitze'; she steps up to her bed and mentions the good hours in the beginning and the difficult hours later on, and then she lights a small candle on the bedside table and places it into a elongated, sand-filled bowl at the foot of the bed. Sieglinde does the same. Victoria [administrative staff] and myself just say 'I wish you a good journey', which was the phrase Tanja and Sieglinde had ended with. Everybody also lights a candle and places it in the bowl. Then it is the relatives' turn, the brother says something in Hebrew, we will later wonder whether Mrs Spitze might have been Jewish. Towards the end of the ceremony Tanja gets all nervous, because she has the impression there are not enough candles for the relatives, but that is not the case, there are enough. She whispers and radiates nervousness, which I find lacks a bit of respect. Then we leave the relatives alone in the room, without saying much more, the brother is visibly moved, and we go our professional ways.

For some time thereafter, I assumed that this was the standard form of the Ritual. That impression persisted because, in the beginning of my fieldwork, I did not usually attend the Ritual. This was because I still felt quite distant from most patients and did not want to intrude. Both personally and in my role as ethnographer I was also shy about engaging in apparently spiritual practices that I did not believe in.

After a while, once I had lost my initial inhibitions, I realised that the Ritual was much less of a clearly defined institution than I had thought. On the one hand, it turned out that it was more individually assembled than I had assumed, often improvised, and sometimes combined diverse elements to a degree that made the whole arrangement seem artificial. On the other hand, it became increasingly clear to me that the ritual was contested and that not all nurses agreed with practising it at all. The following narrative recounts the time when I first realised both these aspects:

A Mrs Dahlberg has died, I have never seen her. On the desk [in the staff room] is an open file, in it a list with the heading 'Farewell Rituals'. Under the first subheading, 'General points', components and functions of rituals are listed; it is not really anthropological, but not popular knowledge either, seems a bit psychotherapeutic to me, 'let's assemble a ritual to help us in difficult times' type-of-thing. I can well imagine a weekend seminar for such a topic, in which rituals are discussed. Under a second subheading, a few short rules for rituals at Stadtwald Hospice are listed, quite general really, no practical guidelines there.

It appeared from my brief reading of the file that the Ritual was in many ways a reflexively planned, almost postmodern ritual, assembled from popularised anthropological and psychotherapeutic sources, and very malleable and adaptable to those circumstances when it was perceived there was 'something to work on' in this way. My diary text continues:

... Later, someone asks me whether I would like to participate in the Ritual for Mrs Dahlberg; I say no, I have never seen her. Greta also does not participate, neither does Theresa. After my refusal I look to Greta for affirmation, and ask again, she says, yes, that's OK, one does not have to participate. What, does one not any more, Theresa looks up and asks, no, says Greta decidedly, one does not. My impression that the Ritual is not very popular is again strengthened.

It turned out with time that some nurses in fact resented the Ritual and never participated. The above text suggests ('not any more') that there had indeed been an obligation to participate which had then been lifted. Other nurses were greatly in favour of the Ritual, volunteered for its preparation, and always tried to make time available for it. There were, in one or two instances, discussions in whose shift this time-consuming procedure was to take place, and I could not help the impression that these were in fact veiled discussions about its overall importance.

With time I also realised that the Ritual did, in fact, not have a fixed form, as I had initially thought. Rather, the people who prepared it tried to choose a form which they thought was appropriate to the biography and spiritual outlook of the patient in question. The candle procedure I had first witnessed was but one possible form, if apparently a frequent one, especially when nurses were pressed for time. There were other possibilities, though. I attended one Ritual of an old woman who had been Roman Catholic, and the nurse in charge had selected a Christian prayer to be read and two church songs, which we sang. Some lines were said about what was known about her life, as was customary in many such Rituals.

Another time, Riccarda, a patient with schizophrenia, who the nurses liked very much, had died. The nurse in charge told me in great detail during an interview how her Ritual had been conducted: Riccarda, who had liked colourful clothes, was dressed in her favourite clothing. Nurses made up her face and painted her nails as she had usually done herself. Her cigarettes – she had been a chain smoker – were placed on her body, together with her favourite handbag. The Ritual then included the reading of a Buddhist mantra, the playing of a tape recording of a sad song by a popular German entertainer, and the reading of a short story. Two nurses stayed in the room for some time afterwards, smoked cigarettes and told each other stories they remembered of Riccarda. One of them told me in an interview that Riccarda had been a colourful person and that she had played many roles in her life as a schizophrenic, so the way to remember her ought to be colourful and varied. While some of the nurses remembered this Ritual as a particular well suited one, the undertakers were, as I was told, slightly puzzled by the unusual sight when they came.

However, even once I had become quite familiar with Stadtwald Hospice, I never quite figured out how frequently Rituals took place and how important they really were for staff members. It seemed to me that there were rather few Rituals considering the number of patients who died and that they rarely took on elaborate forms as in Riccarda's case. I concluded that a large, but silent group of the nurses did not support the Ritual actively and tried to avoid organising one, while a more vociferous group, maybe a minority, saw it as an indispensable part of hospice ways.

In any case, Rituals were only conducted for patients who had been at the hospice for some time and whom at least some nurses had liked. This points, in fact, to their social function, which has not been discussed so far. The Ritual – as its alternative name, 'The Farewell' [Ger.: Die Verabschiedung], also shows – ended the nurse-patient relationship, and the nurses were clearly aware of that function. 'A good ritual', said the nurse in the interview mentioned above, 'gives us strength and ends the nursing situation. When we clean up the room afterwards, it's not the patient any more.'

The Ritual, as discussed so far, was assembled, contested and possibly infrequent. However, the analysis links up in several ways with hospice practice as analysed in previous chapters: first of all, the fact that there were written yet flexible guidelines, apparently adapted for the purpose from anthropological or psychological sources, points back to the reflexivity and openness of the institutional atmosphere mentioned in chapter one. Furthermore, the general form of the Ritual, flexible to the point of almost not being recognisable, made it patient-centred in the extreme. Very diverse biographic and spiritual references – mainly those of the patients, but always through the eyes of the nurses – could thus be accommodated. Indeed, the importance of biography and individual preferences in the Ritual is again in line with the reflexive, individualist self-projects discussed in the previous chapters of this study, and with hospice staff's determination to prolong such projects as much as possible.

Finally, the question reoccurs of to what extent such reflexive projects were really those of the patients and to what extent they originated with the nurses. In the case of the Ritual, it can clearly be seen that typical assumptions of self, as discussed previously, continued to be of importance to the nurses even once the patient in question was dead. It thus originated with the nurses in this case. What gave those who celebrated the Ritual the strength the one nurse mentioned can be interpreted as a celebration of individualist biography composition, communally achieved in the end, and emphasised even after death.

However, the nursing relationship was terminated by the Ritual, or another form of more individual farewell. There was no communal vision into what kind of state the deceased would be reintegrated and by what means. The Ritual was, in my opinion, more of an elaborate personal greeting than a classical rite of passage. It owed its character on each occasion to the nature and strength of the social bonds ended by it, which it broke off so that cleaning staff and undertakers could take over.

The farewell situation and attitudes towards grief in general are a suitable point to come back to the assertion made in chapter two, that much of the emotionality at the hospice was professional and mostly one-sided. The amount of emotions displayed by staff when somebody died was not uniform and, as should be expected, depended on the type of relationship that had formed with a patient. However, mostly there was no display of grief. Respect and compassion played a great role, feelings of relief that suffering had ended were often expressed, but grief, at least public grief, was very rare amongst staff. One nurse told me that she had cried once since she was employed at Stadtwald Hospice, when the hospice's very first patient died, and never again after.

However, in some cases stronger relationships formed, especially when patients stayed at the hospice for a very long time, as Mrs Pietsch did, an unassuming, working-class woman of about ninety years who remained at Stadtwald Hospice for almost a year. When she died, the story of her life was mentioned at handover – a great exception from normal handover procedure:

> At handover at the end of the shift we start at the top end [of the main corridor], number one – Mr Bohnert, number two – Mr Müller, ... and when we get to Mrs Pietsch – number 11, Caroline briefly looks up to Klara, but after a moment says herself, Mrs Pietsch died last night at ten past one, the son was there, the other one came this morning... and continues to talk about the usual stuff, undertaker, inheritance, smart card [of the insurance company], ID card, and so on. Has the Farewell already taken place? No, we have all done that by ourselves, says Caroline. So have I during the shift. Somebody asks how long she has been here, since 20th March – I notice that she knows the exact date. When she has finished Hartmut says he talked to the son yesterday, the one from Munich, and learned something about the very difficult life of Mrs Pietsch, how she had to struggle a lot, that she had a very difficult relationship with her parents, how protection had been an issue, it played an important role. Protection she received, somebody asks, no, which she often gave others, you would not have thought that of the fragile little woman. Hartmut talks softly as usual, but also in a determined way; this is important to him, I think. Caroline says yes, she had heard that from the son, she knew. Nobody says what exactly is meant. It does not really matter, either. Well, little Mrs Pietsch, says Maria, and it seems to me she has tears in her eyes. A very long pause follows, until Caroline says, OK, number 12 – Mrs Berger. I am very touched: I have a feeling as if Mrs Pietsch had been especially honoured, since I have been here nobody has been remembered at handover in such a way before, in passing of course, but still quite moving from the point of view of somebody who works here.

Chapter three has introduced the point that stories are about departures from the ordinary. The story above is once again about such a breach of a routine, a breach which seemed extraordinary to me and thus made it into my diaries: while discussing patients at handover, room after room, suddenly there was an unusually personal display of emotions about the death of Mrs Pietsch. In fact, the narrative about her death opens with the standard things said at such occasions, the standard narrative pattern to follow: died at such and such a time, arrangement with undertakers, arrangement with doctor, arrangement with relatives. But then, quite suddenly, there was something like a short commemoration of her person

106

and her life within the standard handover procedure, until we went on to the next room, the next patient, and thus re-established standard routine.

It was my impression that stronger emotional bonds, such as with Mrs Pietsch, were formed mostly with patients who did not quite fit the ideas of self discussed at length before: staff reacted with greatest sadness to the deaths of some patients who had been at Stadtwald Hospice for a long time, who were simple in their outlook, who did not verbalise their situation and their life a lot and who had just been there in their often idiosyncratic ways. Maybe it was the case that another, unreflexive life world had sneaked in and taken staff by surprise, as if an old relative had suddenly died. In such cases, which remained rare, the card announcing a patient's funeral or cremation was put on the board in the staff room instead of the one in the entrance hall usually reserved for such cards, and staff members sometimes went to the funerals of such patients.

When the body was prepared and all farewells said, the undertakers would usually take the patient away within a day at the most. The relationship between hospice staff and the undertakers, who came to take the bodies of deceased patients away, was uneasy. The undertakers usually came from many different companies, frequently from different parts of the country. They were often quite rough, hands-on men whose job was really about carrying coffins and driving vans, and whose demeanour resembled that of builders or mechanics rather than that of the caring professions. The coffin which they brought with them often almost clogged up the hospice corridor, an unintended but fitting symbolism. Hospice staff attributed little importance to the undertakers' work, but many were quick to point out their lack of manners, punctuality and respect for the dead.[4]

In one handover, this came to light in a struggle over whether the Ritual of a dead person or the undertakers' wish to take them away was to be more important:

I am on the shift with Greta and Laura, Werner also arrives shortly before handover, so we are well staffed with experienced people. Mrs Haussmann has died, I notice by the candle on the corridor. Guido does the handover for her, and mentions that the 'Ritual' is still to be carried out. In the middle of handover, the undertaker arrives. 'Sorry for disturbing your lunch break', he says, apparently not realising that what he finds is the opposite of a lunch break, rather one of the most important components of the shift. In a very stern fashion Mario says, you have been scheduled for 3.30 pm; it is not possible now, a farewell still has to be carried out. The others support him strongly. Whether it could not be done a little earlier, the undertaker asks, Mario says no, he should go and 'fetch somebody else' in the meantime. Do you know where I come from, the undertaker says, from Bochum. You know, goes Kerstin, why don't you go over to the kitchen, you will get a coffee there, and thus ends the discussion. The undertaker still adds, well, maybe a few minutes earlier would be possible, and then leaves. We are not going to give in to that, Kerstin says, Guido mutters something like, great, a ritual under time pressure. I have a feeling as if the undertaker has come up against a brick wall, and while writing down this anecdote that impression intensifies.

The undertaker in question, probably misled by the apparently casual hospice atmosphere, not knowing what a handover and a Ritual were and how crucially important good timing was in nursing work ethics, met with no sympathy whatsoever from hospice staff. Not even an attempt was made to explain to him why he could not proceed as he wished, and a veritable clash of workplace cultures ensued. All this was of course in striking contrast to the understanding behaviour nurses displayed towards patients, relatives and visitors. The undertakers were clearly part of another world, the practices and values of which had hardly anything in common with the world of hospice nursing, and they were treated accordingly.

Once the undertakers had gone and taken the body away, commemoration of patients who had died took several forms: there was a book, always on display outside the staff room, into which patients' names and the dates of their deaths were entered. A small, red origami star would then be hung from the ceiling of the ward, where there were thus quite a number of origami stars. A card would be written to relatives a year after a patient's death, and there was a yearly interfaith service to commemorate former patients of the hospice. However, except for the service, all this was done mostly as a matter of administrative routine – the hospice's area of competence, at least concerning patients, ended in stages: with death, with the Farewell, and with the taking away of a patient's corpse. In the practical world of hospice life, the patient was usually replaced by a living patient with new characteristics the following day.

Commemorating the dead was a fixed point on the hospice agenda, but in terms of time and other resources not a very significant one at all. This is the only point where my own ethnographic experience concerning treatment of the dead differs significantly from the findings of Christine Pfeffer, who writes that commemoration was a very prominent practice in the hospice she studied, and that social death was to be prevented there even after biological death (Pfeffer 1998: 153–57).

Narrative Patterns Surrounding Death

Amongst staff there were a number of recurring narrative patterns around the topic of death. Especially the exact point in time of somebody's death and the circumstances influencing it were the subject of stories which were told more than once and seemed to be part of a certain repertoire. The most widely circulated kind of these stories centred on the importance of the presence or absence of loved ones for the timing of death. A typical example is the following:

> During the last couple of days of her life, Mrs Gruhl gets thinner and thinner in an unbelievable way. When she arrived four weeks ago she was already a tiny, extremely skinny person, but now one can see every bone, she seems like a skeleton, almost a

mummy. During the last three days she stops eating, only drinks millilitres from a syringe, and finally spends more than a day without any intake of food or fluid. She dies in the presence of her friend 'Mausi' [Ger. diminutive for mouse] and her-daughter-in law. The nurses notice with astonishment how Mrs Gruhl keeps herself alive on the most economical of levels during the last days, and one says she has been waiting for Mausi – who really comes back from a holiday on the day of her death – in order to die. In the nurses' tales it is a matter of course that the presence or absence of certain people has a clear influence on the timing of death, even for those patients who are not conscious any more.

The plot of this story, namely that death, even though physical symptoms made it seem imminent, was only possible for someone in the presence of certain people, was quite common. For many nurses, it was a matter of fact that even unconscious people sometimes waited for important others to visit before they died. More precisely, it was most often emotional matters that were said to hold up or accelerate death. A closely related version of the storyline described above was a bit less common, but also told a number of times: it mentioned patients who had been cared for by their relatives 24 hours a day and who had died alone in the five minutes when somebody had left the room, e.g. to go to the toilet. It was then said that such patients needed to be alone. In both types of stories, it was assumed that patients always sensed the presence of others and had some sort of intentionality in choosing the moment of their own death.

In the case of one patient, Mrs Spitze, whose Ritual was described above, a similar story was told, the difference being that this time, the patient herself apparently felt that her death was foreshadowed by the stopping of her watch and that she was then held back by the visit of relatives she did not like:

Tanja, who in any case tells lots of tales, tells one about Mrs Spitze, saying that she wanted to die. Her watch had stopped, and that gave her hope, because her husband's watch had also stopped two days before his death. Sometimes her brother comes on unexpected visits, 'we want to surprise her', and is not very welcome. On the last day Maria sends him away, having asked Mrs Spitze, who wants it that way. The brother has to go, his wife too. Afterwards Tanja says that Mrs Spitze was very upset; her brother had kept her from dying.

Again, emotions were seen to be central by the patient and the nurse, this time dislike of the patient's brother and probably unfinished personal business with him.

A similar type of intentionality and choice was displayed in some stories that were told about patients who chose to give up. I remember one patient, whom his doctor had told he had only about three more months to live, died within two weeks after this disclosure. Similar stories had been told to me before. This type of pattern, again shedding some light on issues of being informed or not, was called 'turning to the wall' by the nurses, and also related in stories a couple of times. 'After x or y had happened, he just turned to the wall and died' was the outline of the plot of such stories. It again implied that people had a considerable degree of influence over the moment of their death and again emotions were seen to be central; this time absence of hope and resulting loss of courage and faith in life.

I once had a conversation about this with one nurse, who in the spectrum of hospice nurses was more on the biomedical side and normally had a marked impatience for ritual practices and what she considered superstition. In her view, she pointed out, a typology of how people died was to some extent possible according to their personality types:

> She says there is a type of man who does not like to be touched and caressed by the nurses, friendly conversation, yes, but no physical contact. This type then does not really get confined to bed, but dies suddenly and almost standing. In fact, it had once happened to her that one such man got up, sat down in the chair and died there. Apparently she sympathises with these men. Her account touches me, because it fits some people I met here: Mr Müller, and the railway worker, I forget his name, and in parts also Mr Bullinger. Maybe there is a kind of hope for redemption there, one would like to die that way, not in a coma.

The emotionality in question here is more indirect, but still quite clear: those who lived their life without much physically expressed affection or openly displayed emotion, according to this kind of story, preferred to die while still independent, and indeed managed to do so. Not insignificantly, the nurse who told the story was herself a very independent, rational and sober woman who would probably not have minded dying standing herself.

I cannot judge from experience whether such behavioural patterns in patients were really frequent. Whatever the case may be, the above text, the personality of the nurse who told it to me and my own reactions in it, make it apparent that it was not only patients' emotions that were in question: the nurses' fears and hopes about dying played a role in the construction and circulation of such narratives, too. There was, in my opinion, an element of reassurance and hope for them in such stories. After all, nurses saw a lot of deaths, peaceful ones, but also terrible ones, and it is understandable that the thought of one's own death and its circumstances comes up through such exposure. This is also shown in the following text:

> During the night Mrs Ohler died, two rooms are empty now. Mrs Ohler's death somehow gives me a calm feeling, up to two or three days before her death she preserved her mobility in a wheelchair, smoked and sat in the kitchen. I remember her indecent jokes, which she cracked on the terrace a couple of weeks ago. Then, I am told, she apparently just stayed in bed one day, stopped eating, and died after being bedridden for two days. It does happen without long agony.

The short narrative portrays my own relief that death-defying behaviour – sexual innuendo, smoking, mobility – can continue until right to the end of life, and that only a very short and peaceful 'dying' phase came before the end. In contrast, horrifying deaths occurred as well, not often, but regularly. These were hardly ever passed on in circulated narratives at all.

There is a link here to the function of narratives discussed in detail in earlier chapters, to their particular suitability for non-hierarchical, liberal contexts: at the hospice, there was no institutional guideline as to how nurses were to deal with death on an individual, private level. Some were religious, others atheist, some believed psychotherapy would help people in dealing with death, others practised yoga or reiki to relax in times of professional tension. All were encouraged to think about their feelings and attitudes, but no conclusions were forced, or even suggested. Nurses insisted very much on their own autonomy in expressing themselves and dealing with their own emotions. Significantly, it had been difficult to establish regular psychological supervision at the hospice. While there were some supervision sessions, these were limited to the discussion of certain cases of patients whose behaviour made them problematic for the running of the hospice. To speak the self into discourse in a therapeutic way was, after all, not a common practice amongst nurses. In line with my earlier discussion of the role of narratives in hospice life, I suggest that stories of well-timed death, because of their open and underdetermined nature, were particularly well suited to provide some indirect reassurance in an environment where no direct, universally valid rules applied. In this function, however, they were something of an undercurrent, important for some nurses, maybe not for others.

In addition, the notion of a possibility of timing death fits holistic hospice ideas of body and person, as discussed in chapter three under the heading of 'fading life': This is best explained by pointing out that the contrasting concept – total inability of a person to influence the point of their death – owes itself to the biomedical understanding of the body as a sophisticated physiological machine, over the internal running and failing of which the will or the emotions have at the most very indirect power. Once this dualistic concept is abandoned, the idea that the will or the emotions could influence the body very significantly suggests itself readily. The concept of timed death is thus in accordance with the hospice understanding of body and person, and stories of timed death suit the institutional atmosphere of the hospice well as an indirect device of reassurance for those nurses who need it.

Notes

1. My ethnographic account here mostly confirms the findings of Pfeffer (1998: 113–56), but ultimately differs in the description and interpretation of social death and remembrance after death.

2. There is a vast and sophisticated anthropological literature on actual death and associated practices in many societies around the globe. There are three central, related concerns in most such studies: first, rites of passage (van Gennep 1986[1909]), applied e.g. by Glaser and Strauss (1965b); second, burial and surrounding ritual, especially multiple burial (Hertz 1928a); and third, the impact of death on social structure and different kinds of response to it (Bloch and Parry 1982, Huntington and Metcalf 1991[1979], Feldmann 1997). All three themes are only of limited relevance in the present context: burial took place outside the hospice sphere, after the corpse had been taken from the hospice and mostly without hospice involvement. While, at Stadtwald Hospice, there was the passage out of life and rituals associated with it, as will be seen below, these were mainly farewell rituals from the hospice staff point of view. While the notion of liminality in Victor Turner's very broad sense (Turner 2000[1969]) can be applied to the hospice context for a broader sociological analysis (e.g. by Lawton 2000), most criteria normally associated with rites of passage, such as more strictly defined liminal states of mind or re-integration of the dead into other realms of existence, were not very relevant in my research experience. Finally, most patients had been taken out of all but the most immediate social structures long before their death, and the remaining impact of death on families and individual relatives mostly lay beyond the reach of hospice nurses.

3. The practices I witnessed and described in my diaries seemed too varied and irregular to me to warrant a productive application of ritual theory in the stricter sense. Mattingly (1998: 161–66) discusses some relations between ritual and therapeutic emplotment, but I find her presentation inconclusive.

4. For more detail on undertakers in Germany see Hänel (2003).

6
CONCLUSION

⚜

Ethnographic Summary

As a means of introducing the concluding theoretical points of the study, I shall now summarise the material discussed thus far and the conclusions drawn from it. Presenting hospice care in a nutshell, the first chapter started out with a story about a patient, Hans Dornschuh, and myself. I used that story to make clear that at Stadtwald Hospice, where everything was somehow related to death, the focus of my research turned out to be life.

It was then pointed out that the life phase 'dying' somehow mediates between life and death in contemporary Western societies. It rests on biomedical knowledge and authority in a crucial way, requiring a terminal diagnosis in the beginning and a definite point of death in the end. Neither of these two points, especially not notions of biological death, are a natural given outside social conventions. Drawing on the work of Hans Blumenberg, Thomas Macho and James Fernandez, it was suggested that 'death' as a point in time is always a construct, and that 'death' as the antithesis of life can only ever be approximated through metaphoric predication. The term remains an absolute metaphor, designating something which cannot be known directly or defined unequivocally.

It was then explained how the idea of a life-cycle period called 'dying', with its continuous predictive reference to death, was an important precondition for the emergence of the hospice movement. Specifically, a long dying phase poses a particular problem to an individualist ideology of continuous self-reflexive and self-responsible actualisation of biographical projects. Especially social death, the end of all meaningful social exchange often preceding biological death, was interpreted as a threat to such a lifestyle. The hospice idea was presented as an attempt to prevent social death from happening before biological death and to make individual choices and projects feasible for the terminally ill for as long as possible. It rests firmly on values relating to self and person which are prevalent in those societies where hospices were developed.

Social scientists of death and dying are not separate from the values and practices of their societies in general and of those of their chosen field of study in particular. Sociologists, it was pointed out, were important early advocates of the denial-of-death thesis, which portrayed death as a taboo topic and as bereft of dignity and individuality. This thesis was to become a crucial argument in favour of the hospice movement. In more general terms, I pointed out that patient-centred medicine and qualitative research both prioritise individual experience and thus share a common root. Ultimately, 'dying' provides the vantage point for a specific kind of access to people's life world by hospice nurses, palliative doctors, specialised therapists and, finally, social scientists. This observation served as the starting point for the self-reflexive approach of this study.

The second chapter focused on method and made at least partly visible the circumstances of the production of anthropological knowledge in the case of my work. It furnished basic data about the hospice and its integration into the health system. I analysed an institutional atmosphere which, because of media attention and a great turnover of several kinds of short-term visitors, proved to be quite conducive to the start of my fieldwork. It was then shown how an initially relatively broad research interest became increasingly focused in a back-and-forth movement between the topic, the field and the researcher's person and interests.

Guiding ideas of the study changed in the course of my fieldwork: a focus on death was replaced by an interest in life with severe illness, a focus on abstract thought was replaced by a study of everyday practices, and my methodological attention turned from symbolic systems to narrative. The common denominator for these changes was that they all had to do with the movement from outside to inside, with the crossing of two boundaries: the boundary that lies between theoretical anthropology as intellectual activity and concrete participation in fieldwork, and the boundary that lies between the outside representation and the inside practice of hospices. In this way, the changes described are a result of the classical ethnographic process: going there, coming back again, and telling the story. In all the change described, my overarching concern remained the question as to how meaning was constructed in hospice care.

The aim of the third chapter was to take a first ethnographic look at Stadtwald Hospice. It was shown that a strong figurative emphasis on life and on being distinct from other healthcare institutions, as reflected in the layout and decoration of the hospice, had its root in a specific understanding of nursing, prioritising positive lived experience over biomedical therapy as practised in hospitals. The approach could be subsumed under the image of the private household, which was implemented in the hospice in contradistinction to that of the public healthcare institution.

The ethnography then turned to the daily routines of nursing care. I used examples of a very dependent patient, Mr Rathje, and a comparatively independent one, Mrs Mertens, to demonstrate how everyday tasks, such as helping patients to get up, to wash, or to eat, were characterised by an activating attitude which left as many aspects of daily life as possible to the patient to decide. Independence, conscious experience and choice can be seen as central values of hospice care in the diary excerpts presented. In Stadtwald Hospice, it was assumed that even a very ill patient had cognition, intentions and desires hardly different from those of healthy adults, and that she would appreciate as much independence, conscious experience and choice as possible. However, nursing based on such values encountered obstacles when patients were too ill to express themselves. It was shown that communication, to some extent, had to be based on assumptions about the patient.

In more general terms, nurses' ways of dealing with patients aimed at a reconstruction of their social persona by filling in gaps, either through assumptions or through nurses' own actions. In a similar way, patients' physical integrity often had to be reconstructed: bodies were prepared carefully for public presentation in order to conceal stigmatising aspects of cancer and make social interaction possible.

I introduced the notion of fading life in order to illustrate shared aspects of all patients' illness trajectories in the hospice. The case of Mrs Brunnhofer showed how changes in body, mind and personality of patients combined in one process in which such categories themselves were often indistinguishable and in which biomedical and psychosocial causalities became blurred. Life as such faded, and nurses did not perceive patients as cultural or psychological entities placed on a failing body. Subsequently, in the nurses' daily work, there was no clear boundary between nursing tasks and psychosocial care for patients.

Hospice nurses would, within such a framework, put a lot of time and energy into making patients' lives at Stadtwald Hospice more enjoyable and more dignified. This was attempted in particular by encouraging conscious positive experience of everyday situations. Thus, the patients' subjective well-being was enhanced in ways that were probably much less common in other institutions. In most cases, patients' and nurses' views in these matters coincided – patients seemed satisfied with the care they received, and nurses with what they considered a fulfilling professional life in an unusual institution. By the standards of its patients and their relatives, and by its own standards, Stadtwald Hospice was a very successful institution indeed.

However, with patients who wanted less rather than more autonomy and thus did not share core hospice values, misunderstandings could arise: the hospice approach could become problematic with patients who would simply have liked to have strict routines, to surrender their power to decide, and who were maybe not used to making their own choices at all.

Many nurses favoured relationships in which patients' autonomy was used to establish mutuality in daily interaction, and in which one-sided disclosure by the patient in emotional matters prevailed. Most nurses' emotional interest in the patients was limited by clear spatial and temporal boundaries. Still, nurses liked to be an important precondition for patients' positive experience at the hospice and were dissatisfied with one patient, Mr Nolte, who considered their work as merely a service. Staff were prepared to make great efforts to improve patients' situation when patients agreed to cooperation in daily interaction, trust and one-sided emotional disclosure. In addition, the nurses had more information at their disposal than the patients. Thus, even in such a patient-centred environment, nurses ultimately had a clear emotional and informational advantage over patients.

Nurses often considered their work successful when patients experienced daily care as pleasant and felt dignified, comfortable and as independent as possible. However, the decision as to whether an interaction was successful or not was often taken by the nurse, and patients sometimes had only an indirect say in it. It was noted that there was hardly any talk of failure at the hospice, and I attributed this to the flexibility of the patient-centred approach which, in combination with the fading life of patients, meant that the nurses were likely either to find out what a patient exactly wanted, or to have their way anyway due to the patients' declining strength. Until that point, the hospice ethos would frame any conflict as something to be worked on, and doing so was seen as a positive procedure, not a failure.

The first part of the fourth chapter asked how hospice values were put into actual social practice through negotiations between patients and nurses. In the case of Toni Schultz, it was shown that stories functioned as legitimation for past behaviour and suggested standards for future behaviour. They were an especially viable means for the negotiation of social practice since they always remained open for interpretation and thus fitted the patient-centred, liberal hospice ethos better than a more direct, maybe hierarchical way of negotiation and communication. An emphasis on stories as the basis for establishing standards of practice was thus in accordance with hospice values.

I then turned from the function of stories to their content and extended the discussion of the negotiation of hospice life to an analysis of the kind of life that was to be negotiated. Using diary excerpts about Mr Urban, it was shown that self-reliance was to be used to find and overcome obstacles through effort and training, based on identification and acceptance of the limits imposed by fading life. Many nurses made offers of time, care and effort more readily when a patient was willing to take charge of her life. They found those patients most difficult who were demanding without accepting responsibility for themselves. It was noted that, on a practical plane, a clear expression of desires and consciously chosen goals made nurses' daily work easier, too.

The second part of the chapter analysed attempts to construct meaningful experience for patients against the backdrop of fading life. Cheryl Mattingly's notion of therapeutic emplotment was used as a tool in the analysis. It was described how, starting out from pre-discursive nursing actions and rudimentary communication, hospice staff presented to patients a continuous, subtle enticement to engage with the world and to experience the world as meaningful and pleasant in ways that the patients had no longer deemed possible.

Once the patients' desire for such experience was kindled, the staff tried to shape a shared plot in interaction with patients, projecting into the future further desirable ends – another good meal, another pleasant walk – that it could be worth working towards. It was shown how such attempts to emplot shared experience sometimes succeeded, sometimes stopped half-way and sometimes never took off at all. However, in those cases when they succeeded, not only patients, but also staff had meaningful experiences to talk about. Meaning-making was not just for the benefit of one side. In the final example of Mr Kasparek, I tried to widen the perspective and to picture emplotment as a pervasive attitude, an approach to body and personality in actions and communication, rather than a distinct, tool-like strategy.

Emplotting clinical time into narrative time and crystallising passing events into worthwhile experience was a crucial, underlying goal of hospice nursing. The goals and normative assumptions lie in the apparent openness of such an attitude. The nurses were not primarily interested in influencing the content of a given patient's experience, but in whether she had a significant experience at all. The normative level of hospice care as a patient-centred approach to nursing was found not so much in prescriptive behaviour towards patients' lives but in guiding assumptions about the patients' self, upon which an ethos of conscious experience and self-actualisation was based. Thus, any significant experience could be classed as good experience from the hospice point of view.

Anything else only left a blank. I concluded that one reason for the absence of accounts of failure was that the hospice idea of success – any experience worth relating – coincided with general structural requirements for stories to be told. No experience: no story to tell: no failure to talk about. In the patient-centred discourse about experience, anything that did not produce a story could not be represented. Successfully facilitating experience and having stories to talk about were two aspects of the same set of practices, hospice nursing.

At Stadtwald Hospice, in conclusion, there was no rigid prescription as to what kind of life a patient had to lead. Approaches depended decisively on patients' personalities, backgrounds and individual illness trajectories. There was considerable institutional leeway in structuring patients' lives and nurses' approaches to their work. There was, however, a clear assumption of self, prestructuring what kind of life a patient was encouraged to lead. It was based on an aware, active self, engaging with the situation of fading life, confiding emotionally in the nurses and cooperating with them in the construction of everyday tasks as pleasant and meaningful, through training and effort if necessary.

The last ethnographic chapter took a closer look at actual deaths at Stadtwald Hospice and at the social and cultural arrangements surrounding them. The chapter started with a discussion of the signs which the nurses interpreted as heralding impending death. It was noted that the actual 'dying' phase at the hospice was very short and patients were only considered as 'dying' in the very last days or even hours of their lives. Care arrangements during that phase were described, and it was demonstrated how hospice staff tried to spend a lot of time both with dying patients and with their relatives.

After death, the bodies of deceased patients were carefully prepared for relatives and nurses to say farewell. The farewell ceremony called the 'Ritual' at the hospice was analysed as a reflexively planned ritual inspired by popularised social science sources and assembled from texts, songs or other material from patients' lives or nurses' own background. It had little fixed form and offered a lot of space to accommodate individual biographic or spiritual references. I interpreted the Ritual as a form of last greeting which ended the nurse–patient relationship and took the form of a celebration of individual biographies. Amongst the nurses, the Ritual was contested. Whether it took place after a patient's death depended on the strength of the relationships formed, and some nurses never participated. It was noted, however, that the Ritual, as an open, patient-centred, self-reflexive and biographically oriented social arrangement, fit several aspects of hospice atmosphere and ethos, as analysed in previous chapters, very well.

After the nurse–patient relationship had thus ended, little remained to be done. There were hardly any displays of grief by hospice nurses. In a similar vein, commemorating the dead was, on the one hand, a fixed point on the hospice agenda, but, on the other hand, took up rather little space in the actual everyday life there. It was done in an almost administrative way through postcards and book-keeping. The undertakers who came for the corpses of the deceased patients were considered quite alien to the hospice atmosphere and approaches, a fact which became apparent through frequent misunderstandings between them and members of full-time staff.

At Stadtwald Hospice, there were a number of narrative patterns about hospice death, stories with similar plot lines which were told repeatedly. They typically claimed that patients had a degree of influence over the timing of their deaths, and this was always portrayed as being in some way based on emotions, grounded in hope, affection, or the like. I interpreted this finding as congruent with the holistic hospice understanding of body and person, where emotions were seen as being able to influence the body profoundly. I also suggested that such stories had a reassuring function for the nurses, suggesting a certain amount of control over death.

Theoretical Suggestions

The Construction of Life

On the basis of the above summary and bearing in mind the typical interplay between specificity and generality that characterises ethnographic knowledge, my concluding theoretical suggestions pertain to the construction of life and the conceptualisation of death. My first point is that hospice nursing can serve as an exemplary and detailed case study in how the cultural life world is constructed in social interaction.[1] This is because, when life fades, every aspect of that world is at stake and demands attention from the hospice point of view.

The (re)construction of the person in hospice nursing could first be seen to encompass the physical level and the construction of bodily appearances.[2] When patients are fed, washed or shaved, when nurses bandage their open wounds or help them to manage their incontinence, the substance and boundaries of the body are regulated in order to meet cultural norms. Nurses fill in the gaps left by bodily changes and the loss of physical abilities. In many cases, material objects like incontinence pads, catheters or wheelchairs take over bodily functions which are no longer available.

When the body can at least partially be brought in line with cultural expectations, hospice nursing tries to build mobility and social contacts on the base thus established. It attempts to enable patients to interact with the world outside the confines of their beds, to be in different places with diverse people. In this area, the fading of life again makes it necessary to fill in gaps, to make use of personal assistance or physical props. Even the social contacts themselves – nurses, volunteers or other patients – can in some cases be seen as placeholders for social contacts that have been lost in the process of fading life.

Similar observations apply to communication. At several points in this study, it could be shown how a social persona is constructed in communication with patients, even when some of the answers or reactions in such communication have to be assumed by the nurses, or detected from very small hints. In hospice nursing, the assumptions and attributions that are made about others in any human communication are applied in at times extreme ways, because fading life often leaves large gaps in the patients' abilities to communicate as well.

Finally, the most culturally specific aspect of the construction of a life world against the backdrop of fading life was the way in which patients were encouraged to adopt specific attitudes towards the use of their remaining time – the socially acceptable use of this time being endangered like any other aspect of life. As has been shown, the idea of the person on which many hospice activities were based and the values which were prominent – such as independence, awareness and choice – were congruent with dominant trends in the societies where hospices originated and successfully developed. In hospice nursing, this meant that, at times, there were subtle pressures to conform to such values, and some behaviours made it easier for nurses to dispense time, energy and emotions than did others.

All the reconstructions described are necessarily precarious and interactive. This fact corresponds neatly with observations made about stories and emplotment in chapter four, namely that stories are underdetermined and emplotment is a social achievement always in danger of collapsing. It is no coincidence, then, that stories prove to be a useful vantage point for inquiry into hospice life. Emplotment, the attempt to build interactive stories and project them into the future, is a strategy of configuring time and structuring experience which potentially links all the levels of reconstruction mentioned, from the most basic physical needs to the most sophisticated attempts to make sense of life, in a narrative format. It suits the field of inquiry for the same reason stories do, in that it is congruent, as a level of analysis and representation, with hospice attitudes and practices.

The Conceptualisation of Death

I have mentioned very early on that, during my fieldwork, I became intriguingly aware that what I was really moving towards was an ethnography of nursing and severe illness. Once I had intellectually understood 'death' as a metaphorical usage and deconstructed 'dying' as quite an artificial notion sometimes far removed from daily life in the hospice, I was left with a field in which all seemed to be legitimated by death and leading to death, but only life could be researched. To conclude my study, I now propose to examine the thesis that, in an often materialist, rationalist and self-reflexive social context, a varied, but intense concern with 'dying', as witnessed in hospice care, is an important contemporary practice of dealing with death itself through various forms of conceptualisation and narrativisation.

At the root of this idea is the initial discussion of the designation 'death' as a metaphor, which substitutes for something that cannot possibly be known directly or defined clearly; only an indirect knowledge of the meaning of 'death' is possible. One way to gain such indirect knowledge is through looking at where the designation appears in language and social life and how it is used there. While this has already been demonstrated for death metaphors by Thomas Macho (1987), I would argue that Macho's understanding of metaphor can be extended to the narratives we tell about dying.

Many metaphors, in fact, necessarily contain narrative or give rise to it; in Carrither's (in press) terms, they are 'story seeds'. I argue that, because of its cognitive inaccessibility, this is especially and significantly true for death; it is a story seed par excellence, the one in which most stories about dying really have their origin. The narratives presented and analysed in this study can thus be understood as extended metaphors, used in social life to encircle death and approximate its meaning, and this understanding, I would argue, has a much more general social dimension: while we have little to say about death itself in contemporary modern societies and superficially accept it, we still cannot help having to face it and get to terms with it. This is why we end up saying all the more about dying, deploring its supposed neglect and telling so many stories about it. Death may be silent for us, but dying still occasions highly creative practices and rich narratives.

In this sense, the life phase called 'dying' has a social function not only in actually establishing new nursing practices required as a consequence of biomedical advances and described in detail in previous chapters, but also by enabling people to come up with new metaphoric and narrative approximations of death, approximations which indirectly supplement the sober biomedical explanations prevalent today. If meaning-making, as Fernandez (1986) argues, is about being moved through metaphoric predication and finding persuasive stories, 'dying' and the hospice movement are one important place where such metaphors and stories can be created, a laboratory for finding new ways of dealing with mortality and with the intellectually elusive meaning of death.

Elisabeth Kübler-Ross's popular account of the dying phases (Kübler-Ross 1969) is one good example for this claim. It is a narrative pattern organised around the root metaphor of death as the crucial point in a journey that potentially leads towards peace and spiritual fulfilment. The individual stories that fit that pattern could not be told without the prerequisite of a life phase called 'dying'. They meet all requirements for a story given in chapter four, and death is presented in them as a secular, yet potentially almost religiously fulfilling, goal. It almost seems that the hope for redemption, once directed towards the afterlife, is now invested into the idealised and much studied dying phase. This leaves biomedical explanations untouched and yet retains all the spiritual functions of older religious narratives.

Furthermore, I would argue that the emergence and resilience of denial theories also have their roots in the metaphorical nature of death in this sense. First of all, it is easy to claim 'denial' when the phenomenon in question is pervasive, yet by definition inaccessible and only ever to be pinned down metaphorically. Second, the denial-of-death thesis so vividly discussed in academia until the 1990s quite possibly has a dimension well beyond its alleged topic. At least as much as being about shortcomings in nursing and medicine, it was about establishing the field of 'dying' – talking about it, institutionalising it in hospices, and the like – as a central reference point and meaning-making practice in relation to death. If death as the opposite of life has no understandable meaning, and death as a point in time rests on social conventions, at least dying can be labelled 'heroic', or 'natural', or the like. Where death cannot be accessed, dying can be. In such an understanding, however, the most disturbing event that can happen is social death: the disappearance of the person who is 'dying'. Social death reappears here in a very broad sense, and by a very different line of argument I come back to the initial claim that this was really what the hospice movement was about.[3]

The peculiar affinity of contemporary meaning-making movements – be they of the existentialist, esoteric, psychotherapeutic, Westernised Tibetan Buddhist, or near- death experience variety – with death, then, has a similar root. Since the reference of the empty metaphor 'death' is always uncertain, it can be developed and extended into very diverse narratives, and since death is still a central aspect of human experience, these narratives can become invested with great rhetorical power. Death is then used, almost in a type of reversed theodicy, to ground mean-ing-making somewhere beyond the reaches of rationalism and the natural science paradigm of the world. Death is invoked as the inexplicable, yet all powerful last metaphysical resort, the ultimate legitimation. The metaphorical nature of the term death is essential for the narratives which are employed to achieve such ends, and dying is their crucial starting point.[4]

Similarly, however, the often competing narratives of the social sciences frame death sometimes in numbers and 'hard facts', sometimes in the subjective stories of interviews and participant observation, and sometimes in promises of secular salvation by meaningful dying and peaceful death. All scholarly statements in the 'social sciences of death and dying' chose their own style of narrativisation.[5] The reflexivity claimed in chapter two of this study is thus brought full circle and another perspective can be gained on the initial claim that the social sciences are deeply involved with their subject matter, in this case death and dying.

Seen in such a light, my own ethnographic study can itself be read as one anthropologist's attempt to surround and encircle death by looking at dying and telling others about it. The result is situated knowledge, located within the socially constitutive configuration from which it was selected by the ethnogra-pher, in the latter's own personality, and in the judgement of the readership. All of these dimensions are intimately socially related – a relationship partly made vis-ible by its reflexive presentation. As has been mentioned previously, narrative ethnography has clear limitations when it comes to representing those social facts that cannot easily be captured in a plot structure. However, as I believe to have demonstrated, a focus on narrative and metaphor lends itself particularly well to studying aspects of meaning and experience in human life and to examining how they are made available and negotiated intersubjectively. Narrative ethnography accommodates reflexivity without becoming too theoretical or excessively self-indulgent, and it has been shown to be especially useful in discussing death and dying. The validity of any narrative, and this one is no exception, ultimately depends to no small degree on its persuasiveness for the reader.

Notes

1. As I pointed out before, I do not wish to imply a far-reaching, constructionist, theoretical stance by using this metaphor.
2. In response to an article (Eschenbruch 2005), Christine Pfeffer has rightly pointed out to me how subtle the difference between construction and reconstruction is in the hospice context – the original of what is supposed to be reconstructed is mostly not available.
3. The fact that hospices seem to be able to muster much more public attention and voluntary support than nursing homes for the elderly also points in this direction.
4. Regarding the rhetoric of denial claims, it is interesting to note that I come to a conclusion which is very similar to the position of Feldmann (1997: 39) and Seale (1998), who, however, arrive there with very different methodological and epistemological premises.
5. Attempts at providing a 'sociology (less often: an anthropology) of death' in Western societies, or even a 'thanatology', are still widespread. Clive Seale has quite recently tried to put death at the heart of the sociological enterprise by claiming that all culture is about death – and that all those who disagree are in denial, an idea he ultimately takes from Peter L. Berger (Seale 1998: 11, 70; Berger 1990[1967], passim). I am sceptical of such claims because of their hermeticism and inherent circularity.

BIBLIOGRAPHY

Where translations or later editions have been used, the year of the first publication in the original language appears in brackets.

Albrecht, Gary L. et al. (eds) (2000) *Handbook of Social Studies in Health and Science.* London: Sage.

Ariès, Philippe (1997[1978]) *Geschichte des Todes.* München: dtv.

Armstrong, David (1984) 'The Patient's View', *Social Science and Medicine,* 18(9): 737–44.

——— (1987) 'Silence and Truth in Death and Dying', *Social Science and Medicine,* 24(8): 651–57.

——— (2000) 'Social Theorizing about Health and Illness' in Gary L. Albrecht, et al. (eds) *Handbook of Social Studies in Health and Science.* London: Sage, pp. 24–35.

Arnason, Arnar (1998) 'Feel the Pain: Death, Grief and Bereavement Counselling in the North East of England', unpublished Ph.D. thesis, Durham, U.K.

Aulbert, Eberhard and Detlev Zech (1997) *Lehrbuch der Palliativmedizin.* Stuttgart, New York: Schattauer.

Bauman, Zygmunt (1992) *Mortality, Immortality and Other Life Strategies.* Cambridge: Polity Press.

Berg, Eberhard and Martin Fuchs (eds) (1999[1993]a) *Kultur, soziale Praxis, Text. Die Krise der ethnographischen Repräsentation.* Frankfurt/Main: Suhrkamp.

Berg, Eberhard and Martin Fuchs (1999[1993]b) 'Phänomenologie der Differenz. Reflexionsstufen ethnographischer Repräsentation' in Eberhard Berg and Martin Fuchs (eds) *Kultur, soziale Praxis, Text. Die Krise der ethnographischen Repräsentation.* Frankfurt/Main: Suhrkamp.

Berg, Marc and Annemarie Mol (1998a) 'Differences in Medicine: An Introduction' in Marc Berg and Annemarie Mol (eds) *Differences in Medicine: Unraveling Practices, Techniques and Bodies.* Durham/U.S.A., London: Duke University Press, pp. 1–12.

———— (eds) (1998b) *Differences in Medicine: Unraveling Practices, Techniques and Bodies*. Durham/U.S.A., London: Duke University Press.

Berger, Peter L. (1990[1967]) *The Sacred Canopy: Elements of a Sociological Theory of Religion*. Garden City: Doubleday.

Berger, Peter L. and Richard Lieban (1960) 'Kulturelle Wertstruktur und Bestattungspraktiken in den Vereinigten Staaten', *Kölner Zeitschrift für Soziologie und Sozialpsychologie*, 12(2): 224–36.

Berger, Peter L. and Thomas Luckmann (1966) *The Social Construction of Reality: A Treatise in the Sociology of Knowledge*. Garden City: Doubleday.

Binder, Beate at al. (eds) (2005) *Ort. Arbeit. Körper. Ethnografie Europäischer Modernen*. Münster et al.: Waxmann (Schriftenreihe Museum Europäischer Kulturen 3).

Bloch, Maurice and Jonathan Parry (eds) (1982) *Death and the Regeneration of Life*. Cambridge: Cambridge University Press.

Blumenberg, Hans (1971) 'Beobachtungen an Metaphern', *Archiv für Begriffsgeschichte*, 15(2): 161–214.

———— (1998[1960]) *Paradigmen zu einer Metaphorologie*. Frankfurt/Main: Suhrkamp.

Bourdieu, Pierre ([1999]1993) 'Narzistische Reflexivität und wissenschaftliche Reflexivität' in Eberhard Berg and Martin Fuchs (eds) *Kultur, soziale Praxis, Text. Die Krise der ethnographischen Repräsentation*. Frankfurt/Main: Suhrkamp, pp. 365–74.

Bruner, Jerome (1986) *Actual Minds, Possible Worlds*. Cambridge/U.S.A.: Harvard University Press.

———— (1990) *Acts of Meaning*. Cambridge/U.S.A.: Harvard University Press.

Buckler, Sarah (in press) *Fire in the Dark: Telling Gypsiness in North East England*. Oxford: Berghahn Books.

Bundesarbeitsgemeinschaft Hospiz (ed.) (2004a) *Ambulante Hospizarbeit. Grundlagentexte und Forschungsergebnisse zur Hospiz- und Palliativarbeit – Teil 1*. Wuppertal: Hospiz Verlag (Schriftenreihe der BAG Hospiz V/1).

———— (2004b) *Stationäre Hospizarbeit. Grundlagentexte und Forschungsergebnisse zur Hospiz- und Palliativarbeit – Teil 2*. Wuppertal: Hospiz Verlag (Schriftenreihe der BAG Hospiz V/2).

———— (2004c) *Hospiz schafft Wissen. Dokumentation der Fachtagung der Bundesarbeitsgemeinschaft Hospiz e.V. vom 9. November 2003*. Wuppertal: Hospiz Verlag (Schriftenreihe der BAG Hospiz VI).

Carrithers, Michael (1991) 'Narrativity: Mindreading and Making Societies' in Andrew Whiten (ed.) *Natural Theories of Mind: Evolution, Development and Simulation of Everyday Mind-Reading*. Oxford: Blackwell, pp. 305–17.

———— (1992) *Why Humans Have Culture: Explaining Anthropology and Social Diversity*. Oxford: Oxford University Press.

———— (1995) 'Stories in the Social and Mental Life of People' in Esther Goody (ed.) *Social Intelligence and Interaction: Expressions and Implications of the Social Bias in Human Intelligence*. Cambridge: Cambridge University Press, pp. 261–76.

———— (in press) 'Story Seeds and the Inchoate' in Ivo Strecker and Christian Meyer (eds) *Rhetoric Culture. Theory, History, Exemplars*. Oxford: Berghahn Books.

Clark, David (1991) 'Contradictions in the Developments of New Hospices: A Case Study', *Social Science and Medicine*, 33(9): 995–1004.

—— (ed.) (1993) *The Sociology of Death: Theory, Culture, Practice*. Oxford: Blackwell.

—— (ed.) (2002) *Cicely Saunders – Founder of the Hospice Movement: Selected Letters 1959–1999*. Oxford: Oxford University Press.

Clifford, James and George E. Marcus (eds) (1986) *Writing Culture: The Politics and Poetics of Ethnography*. Berkeley: University of California Press.

Douglas, Mary (2002[1966]) *Purity and Danger: An Analysis of Concepts of Pollution and Taboo. With a New Preface by the Author*. London, New York: Routledge.

Dreßke, Stefan (2005) *Sterben im Hospiz. Der Alltag in einer alternativen Pflegeeinrichtung*. Frankfurt/Main et al.: Campus.

DuBoulay, Shirley (1990[1987]) *Cicely Saunders. Ein Leben für Sterbende*. Innsbruck: Tyrolia.

Ebeling, Hans (ed.) (1979a) *Der Tod in der Moderne*. Königstein: Hain.

—— (1979b) 'Einleitung. Philosophische Thanatologie seit Heidegger' in Hans Ebeling (ed.) *Der Tod in der Moderne*. Königstein: Hain, pp. 11–31.

Elias, Norbert (1985) *The Loneliness of the Dying*. Oxford: Blackwell.

Eschenbruch, Nicholas (2005) 'Krankenpflege im Hospiz. Ethnographische Überlegungen zum Gebrauch greifbarer und weniger greifbarer Artefakte' in Beate Binder et al. (eds) *Ort. Arbeit. Körper. Ethnografie Europäischer Modernen*. Münster et al.: Waxmann (Schriftenreihe Museum Europäischer Kulturen 3), pp. 543–51.

Feifel, Herman (1959) *The Meaning of Death*. New York, London: McGraw-Hill.

Feldmann, Klaus (1997) *Sterben und Tod. Sozialwissenschaftliche Theorien und Forschungsergebnisse*. Opladen: Leske and Budrich.

Feldmann, Klaus and Werner Fuchs-Heinritz (1995a) 'Der Tod als Gegenstand der Soziologie' in Klaus Feldmann and Werner Fuchs-Henritz (eds) *Der Tod ist ein Problem der Lebenden. Beiträge zur Soziologie des Todes*. Frankfurt/Main: Suhrkamp, pp. 7–18.

—— and —— (eds) (1995b) *Der Tod ist ein Problem der Lebenden. Beiträge zur Soziologie des Todes*. Frankfurt/Main: Suhrkamp.

Fernandez, James W. (1986) *Persuasions and Performances: The Play of Tropes in Culture*. Bloomington: Indiana University Press.

Fine, Gary Alan (1993) 'Ten Lies of Ethnography: Moral Dilemmas of Field Research', *Journal of Contemporary Ethnography*, 22(3): 267–94.

Flick, Uwe (1998[1995]) *Qualitative Forschung: Theorie, Methoden, Anwendung in Psychologie und Sozialwissenschaften*. Reinbek: Rowohlt.

Foucault, Michel (1991[1963]) *Die Geburt der Klinik: Eine Archäologie des ärztlichen Blicks*. Frankfurt/Main: Suhrkamp.

Fuchs, Werner (1971) 'Die These von der Verdrängung des Todes', *Frankfurter Hefte*, 26: 177–84.

Gantois Chaban, Michèle C. (2000) *The Life Work of Dr. Elisabeth Kübler-Ross and its Impact on the Death Awareness Movement*. Lewiston: E. Mellen Press.

Geertz, Clifford (1995[1973]) *Dichte Beschreibung: Beiträge zum Verstehen kultureller Systeme*. Frankfurt/Main: Suhrkamp.

Gerstenkorn, Uwe (2004) *Hospizarbeit in Deutschland: Lebenswissen im Angesicht des Todes*. Stuttgart: Kohlhammer.

Giddens, Anthony (1991) *Modernity and Self-Identity: Self and Society in the Late Modern Age.* Cambridge/UK: Polity Press.

Gill, Derek (1984[1981]) *Elisabeth Kübler-Ross: Wie sie wurde, wer sie ist.* Stuttgart: Kreuz Verlag.

Glaser, Barney G. and Anselm L. Strauss (1965a) *Awareness of Dying.* Chicago: Aldine.

―――― and ―――― (1965b) 'Temporal Aspects of Dying as a Non-Scheduled Status Passage', *American Journal of Sociology,* 71(1): 48–59.

―――― and ―――― (1968) *Time for Dying.* Chicago: Aldine.

Goffman, Erving (1959) *The Presentation of Self in Everyday Life.* New York: Doubleday.

―――― (1985[1963]) *Stigma: Notes on the Management of Spoiled Identity.* New York et al.: Prentice Hall.

Good, Byron (1994) *Medicine, Rationality and Experience: An Anthropological Perspective.* Cambridge: Cambridge University Press.

Goody, Esther (ed.) (1995) *Social Intelligence and Interaction: Expressions and Implications of the Social Bias in Human Intelligence.* Cambridge/U.K.: Cambridge University Press.

Gorer, Geoffrey (1955) 'The Pornography of Death', *Encounter,* 5(4): 49–52.

―――― (1965) *Death, Grief and Mourning in Contemporary Britain.* New York: Doubleday.

Greer, David and Vincent Mor (1986) 'An Overview of National Hospice Study Findings', *Journal of Chronic Diseases,* 39(1): 5–7.

Greer, David et al. (1986) 'An Alternative in Terminal Care: Results of the National Hospice Study', *Journal of Chronic Diseases,* 39(1): 9–26.

Greverus, Ina-Maria et al. (eds) (1988) '*Kulturkontakt, Kulturkonflikt: Zur Erfahrung des Fremden – 26. Deutscher Volkskundekongreß in Frankfurt vom 28. September bis 2. Oktober 1987.* Frankfurt/Main: Institut für Kulturanthropologie und Europäische Ethnologie.

Gronemeyer, Reimer et al. (2004) *Helfen am Ende des Lebens: Hospizarbeit und Palliative Care in Europa.* Wuppertal: Hospiz Verlag (Schriftenreihe der BAG Hospiz, VII).

Hacking, Ian (1999) *The Social Construction of What?* Cambridge/U.S.A.: Harvard University Press.

Hänel, Dagmar (2003) *Bestatter im 20. Jahrhundert: Zur kulturellen Praxis eines tabuisierten Berufs.* Münster: Waxmann (Beiträge zur Volkskultur in Nordwestdeutschland 105).

Haraway, Donna (1988) 'Situated Knowledge: the Science Question in Feminism and the Privilege of Partial Perspective', *Feminist Studies,* 14(3): 575–99.

―――― (1997) *Modest_witness@second_millennium. FemaleMan_meets_oncomouse.* New York, London: Routledge.

Heidegger, Martin (2001[1927]): *Sein und Zeit.* Tübingen: Max Niemeyer.

Hertz, Robert (1928a) 'Contribution à une étude sur la représentation collective de la mort' in Hertz, Robert: *Mélanges de sociologie réligieuse et folklore.* Paris: F. Alcan, pp. 1–98.

―――― (1928b) *Mélanges de sociologie réligieuse et folklore.* Paris: F. Alcan.

Hirschauer, Stefan (2001) 'Ethnografisches Schreiben und die Schweigsamkeit des Sozialen. Zu einer Methodologie der Beschreibung', *Zeitschrift für Soziologie,* 30(6): 429–51.

Hockey, Jennifer Lorna (1990) *Experiences of Death: An Anthropological Account.* Edinburgh: Edinburgh University Press.

Holmberg, Christine (2005) *Diagnose Brustkrebs: Eine ethnografische Studie über Krankheit und Krankheitserleben.* Frankfurt/Main: Campus.

Howe, Jürgen (1992) 'Die Phasentheorie des Sterbens von Kübler-Ross' in Jürgen Howe et al. (eds) *Lehrbuch der psychologischen und sozialen Alternswissenschaft,* Band IV. Heidelberg: Asanger, pp. 54–68.

Howe, Jürgen et al. (eds) (1992) *Lehrbuch der psychologischen und sozialen Alternswissenschaft,* Band IV. Heidelberg: Asanger.

Huntington, Richard and Peter Metcalf (eds) (1991[1979]) *Celebrations of Death: The Anthropology of Mortuary Ritual.* Cambridge: Cambridge University Press.

Illich, Ivan (1983[1976]) *Die Nemesis der Medizin: Von den Grenzen des Gesundheitswesens.* Reinbek: Rowohlt.

James, Nicky and David Field (1992) 'The Routinization of Hospice: Charisma and Bureaucratization', *Social Science and Medicine,* 34(12): 1363–75.

Johnson, Ian S. et al. (1990) 'What Do Hospices Do? A Survey of Hospices in the United Kingdom and the Republic of Ireland', *British Medical Journal,* 300(6727): 791–92.

Kan, Sergei (1992) 'Anthropology of Death in the Late 1980s', *Reviews in Anthropology,* 20(4): 283–300.

Kaschuba, Wolfgang (ed.) (1995) *Kulturen – Identitäten – Diskurse. Perspektiven Europäischer Ethnologie.* Berlin: Akademie (Zeithorizonte 1).

Kellehear, Allan (1984) 'Are We a "Death-denying" Society? A Sociological Review', *Social Science and Medicine,* 18(9): 713–23.

Kirschner, Janbernd (1996) *Die Hospizbewegung in Deutschland am Beispiel Recklinghausen.* Frankfurt/Main et al.: Peter Lang.

Klaschik, Eberhard (2000) 'Palliativmedizin – Definitionen und Grundzüge', *Der Internist,* 41(7): 606–11.

Kleinman, Arthur (1988) *The Illness Narratives: Suffering, Healing and the Human Condition.* New York: Basic Books.

Kübler-Ross, Elisabeth (1969) *On Death and Dying.* London: Travistock.

—— (1987[1971]) *Interviews mit Sterbenden.* Stuttgart: Kreuz-Verlag.

Lakoff, George and Mark Johnson (1980) *Metaphors We Live By.* Chicago: University of Chicago Press.

Lawton, Julia (1998) 'Contemporary Hospice Care: The Sequestration of the Unbounded Body and "Dirty Dying"', *Sociology of Health and Illness,* 20(2): 121–43.

—— (2000) *The Dying Process: Patients' Experiences of Palliative Care.* London, New York: Routledge.

—— (2001) 'Gaining and Maintaining Consent. Ethical Concerns Raised in a Study of Dying Patients', *Qualitative Health Research,* 11(5): 693–705.

Lindemann, Gesa (2002) *Die Grenzen des Sozialen: zur sozio-technischen Konstruktion von Leben und Tod in der Intensivmedizin.* München: Fink (Übergänge 48).

Lindner, Rolf (1981) 'Die Angst des Forschers vor dem Feld. Überlegungen zur teilnehmenden Beobachtung als Interaktionsprozeß', *Zeitschrift für Volkskunde,* 77(1): 51–66.

——— (1988) 'Wer wird Ethnograph? Biographische Aspekte der Feldforschung', in Greverus, Ina-Maria et al. (eds) *Kulturkontakt, Kulturkonflikt: Zur Erfahrung des Fremden – 26. Deutscher Volkskundekongreß in Frankfurt vom 28. September bis 2. Oktober 1987.* Frankfurt/Main: Institut für Kulturanthropologie und Europäische Ethnologie, pp. 99–107.

——— (1995) 'Kulturtransfer. Zum Verhältnis von Alltags-, Medien- und Wissenschaftskultur' in Wolfgang Kaschuba (ed.) *Kulturen – Identitäten – Diskurse. Perspektiven Europäischer Ethnologie.* Berlin: Akademie 1995 (Zeithorizonte 1), pp. 31–44.

Lock, Margaret (2000) 'On Dying Twice: Culture, Technology and the Determination of Death' in Margaret Lock and Alan Young (eds) *Living and Working With the New Medical Technologies: Intersections of Inquiry.* Cambridge/U.K.: Cambridge University Press, pp. 233–62.

Lock, Margaret and Alan Young (eds) (2000) *Living and Working With the New Medical Technologies: Intersections of Inquiry.* Cambridge/U.K.: Cambridge University Press.

Lupton, Deborah (2000) 'The Social Construction of Medicine and the Body' in Gary L. Albrecht et al. (eds) *Handbook of Social Studies in Health and Science.* London: Sage, pp. 50–63.

——— (2003[1994]) *Medicine as Culture: Illness, Disease and the Body in Western Societies.* London: Sage.

Macho, Thomas (1987) *Todesmetaphern.* Frankfurt/Main: Suhrkamp.

Mascia-Lees, Frances et al. (1989) 'The Postmodernist Turn in Anthropology: Cautions From a Feminist Perspective', *Signs,* 15(1): 7–33.

Mattingly, Cheryl (1994) 'The Concept of Therapeutic Emplotment', *Social Science and Medicine,* 38(6): 811–22.

——— (1998) *Healing Dramas and Clinical Plots: The Narrative Structure of Experience.* Cambridge/U.K.: Cambridge University Press.

May, Carl (1993) 'Disclosure of Terminal Prognoses in a General Hospital: The Nurses' View', *Journal of Advanced Nursing,* 18(9): 1362–68.

McInerney, Fran (1992) 'Provision of Food and Fluids in Terminal Care: A Sociological Analysis', *Social Science and Medicine,* 34(11): 1271–76.

Mellor, Philip A. (1993) 'Death in High Modernity: The Contemporary Presence and Absence of Death' in David Clark (ed.) *The Sociology of Death: Theory, Culture, Practice.* Oxford: Blackwell, pp. 11–30.

Mellor, Philip A. and Chris Shilling (1993) 'Modernity, Self-identity and the Sequestration of Death', *Sociology,* 27(3): 411–31.

Mitford, Jessica (1963) *The American Way of Death.* New York: Simon and Schuster.

Mulkay, Michael (1993) 'Social Death in Britain' in Clark, David (ed.) *The Sociology of Death: Theory, Culture, Practice.* Oxford: Blackwell, pp. 31–49.

Mulkay, Michael and John Ernst (1991) 'The Changing Profile of Social Death', *Archives européennes de sociologie*, 32(4): 172–96.

Müller, Monika and Martina Kern (2002) 'Übereinstimmungen und Abgrenzungen. Palliativmedizin und Hospizarbeit im Vergleich', *Der Klinikarzt*, 31(9): 262–65.

Nassehi, Armin and Georg Weber (1989) *Tod, Modernität und Gesellschaft. Entwurf einer Theorie der Todesverdrängung*. Opladen: Westdeutscher Verlag.

Ostner, Ilona and Elisabeth Beck-Gernsheim (1979) *Mitmenschlichkeit als Beruf. Eine Analyse des Alltags in der Krankenpflege*. Frankfurt/Main and New York: Campus.

Parsons, Talcott (1951) *The Social System*. New York: The Free Press.

Pfeffer, Christine (1998) *Brücken zwischen Leben und Tod: Eine empirische Untersuchung in einem Hospiz*. Köln: Köppe (Siegener Beiträge zur Soziologie 1).

––––––– (2005) *"Hier wird immer noch besser gestorben als woanders..." Eine Ethnographie stationärer Hospizarbeit*. Bern: Hans Huber.

Pichlmaier, Heinz (1998) 'Entwicklung der Palliativmedizin in Deutschland' in Aulbert, Eberhard et al. (eds.) *Palliativmedizin – Ein ganzheitliches Konzept*. Stuttgart and New York: Schattauer (Beiträge zur Palliativmedizin 1), pp. 1–7.

Rest, Franco (1998[1989]) *Sterbebeistand, Sterbebegleitung, Sterbegeleit*. Stuttgart et al.: Kohlhammer.

Ricoeur, Paul (1981) *Hermeneutics and the Human Sciences: Essays on Language, Action and Interpretation*. Cambridge/U.K.: Cambridge University Press.

Rose, Nikolas (1989) *Governing the Soul: The Shaping of the Private Self*. London: Routledge.

Sabatowski, Rainer (1999) *Palliativmedizin 2000: Stationäre und ambulante Palliativ- und Hospizeinrichtungen in Deutschland*. Köln: Deutsche Gesellschaft zum Studium des Schmerzes e.V.

Salis Gross, Corina (2001) *Der ansteckende Tod: Eine ethnologische Studie zum Sterben im Altersheim*. Frankfurt/Main and New York: Campus.

Schlich, Thomas and Claudia Wiesemann (eds) (2001) *Hirntod: Zur Kulturgeschichte der Todesfeststellung*. Frankfurt/Main: Suhrkamp.

Schneider, Werner (1999a) *"So tot wie nötig, so lebendig wie möglich!" Sterben und Tod in der fortgeschrittenen Moderne. Eine Analyse der öffentlichen Diskussion um den Hirntod in Deutschland*. Münster and Berlin: LIT (Studien zur interdisziplinären Thanatologie 6).

––––––– (1999b) '"Death Is Not the Same Always and Everywhere" – Socio-Cultural Aspects of Brain Death and the Legislation of Organ Transplantation: The Case of Germany', *European Societies*, 1(3): 353–89.

Schröder, Harry et al. (2003) *Palliativstationen und Hospize in Deutschland: Belastungserleben, Bewältigungspotential und Religiosität der Pflegenden*. Wuppertal: Hospiz-Verlag (Schriftenreihe der BAG Hospiz IV).

Seale, Clive (1989) 'What Happens in Hospices: A Review of Research Evidence', *Social Science and Medicine*, 28(6): 551–59.

––––––– (1991) 'Communication and Awareness About Death: A Study of a Random Sample of Dying People', *Social Science and Medicine*, 32(8): 943–52.

––––––– (1995) 'Heroic Death', *Sociology*, 29(4): 597–613.

———— (1998) *Constructing Death: The Sociology of Dying and Bereavement.* Cambridge/U.K.: Cambridge University Press.

Seale, Clive et al. (1997) 'Awareness of Dying: Prevalence, Causes and Consequences', *Social Science and Medicine,* 45(3): 477–84.

Seitz, Oliver and Dieter Seitz (2002) *Die moderne Hospizbewegung in Deutschland auf dem Weg ins öffentliche Bewusstsein: Ursprünge, kontroverse Diskussionen, Perspektiven.* Herbolzheim: Centaurus.

Simpson, Michael A. (1987[1979]) *Dying, Death and Grief: A Critical Bibliography.* Pittsburgh: University of Pittsburgh Press.

Sogyal, Rimpoche (2004) *Das tibetische Buch vom Leben und Sterben. Ein Schlüssel zum tieferen Verständnis von Leben und Tod.* München: Fischer Taschenbuch.

Southard, Samuel (1991) *Death and Dying: A Bibliographical Survey.* New York: Greenwood Press.

Spradley, James P. (1980) *Participant Observation.* New York: Holt, Rinehart and Winston.

Strecker, Ivo and Christian Meyer (eds) (in press) *Rhetoric Culture: Theory, History, Exemplars.* Oxford and New York: Berghahn Books.

Sudnow, David (1967) *Passing On: The Social Organisation of Dying.* Englewood Cliffs: Prentice Hall.

Tedlock, Barbara (1991) 'From Participant Observation to the Observation of Participation: The Emergence of Narrative Ethnography', *Journal of Anthropological Research,* 47(1): 69–93.

Turner, Aaron (2000) 'Embodied Ethnography: Doing Culture', *Social Anthropology,* 8(1): 51–60.

Turner, Victor W. (2000[1969]) *Das Ritual: Struktur und Anti-Struktur.* Frankfurt/Main and New York: Campus.

van Gennep, Arnold (1986[1909]) *Übergangsriten.* Frankfurt/Main: Campus.

Waldenfels, Bernhard (1999) *Vielstimmigkeit der Rede: Studien zur Phänomenologie des Fremden,* Band IV. Frankfurt/Main: Suhrkamp.

Walter, Tony (1991) 'Modern Death: Taboo or Not Taboo', *Sociology,* 25(2): 293–10.

———— (1993) 'Sociologists Never Die: British Sociology and Death' in David Clark (ed.) *The Sociology of Death: Theory, Culture, Practice.* Oxford: Blackwell, pp. 264–95.

———— (1994) *The Revival of Death.* London: Routledge.

Weber, Hans-Joachim (1994) *Der soziale Tod: Zur Soziogenese von Todesbildern.* Frankfurt/Main: Peter Lang.

Wiedenmann, Rainer E. (1992) 'Tod, Kultur und Gesellschaft: Ein Literaturbericht', *Sociologia Internationalis,* 30(2): 117–24.

Whiten, Andrew (ed.) (1991) *Natural Theories of Mind: Evolution, Development and Simulation of Everyday Mind-reading.* Oxford: Blackwell.

INDEX

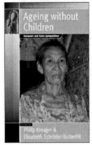